Are You Listening, Doctor?

Are You Listening, Doctor?

Albert Schrut, M.D.

Nelson-Hall nh **Chicago**

All characters in this book are fictional, and any resemblance to persons living or dead is purely coincidental.

Library of Congress Cataloging in Publication Data
Schrut, Albert.
  Are you listening, Doctor?

  1. Psychoanalysis—Case studies. 2. Psychotherapy
patients—Case studies. I. Title.
RC506.S33   616.8'9'09   79-22441
ISBN 0-88229-182-3

Manfactured in the United States of America

10   9   8   7   6   5   4   3   2   1

To Sherry, Judy, Amy, and my mother
and above all, to my patients,
this book is affectionately dedicated

Contents

Chapter 1
Free Associations of a Would-Be Psychiatrist-Psychoanalyst

DR. MILLER: So, Doctor, you find yourself unhappy in general practice after all these years.

Take the couch. Tell me everything you are thinking.

ABE: Why am I, Abraham Sherwood, M.D., on your analytic couch? I've got to find out why I went into medicine and why I'm so disappointed in it. That's why I'm here. Is it because I once thought that as a physician I could see and master all of life? Or is it because I saw myself in every grievous and fearful situation of my patients, and I never knew any of them the way I wanted to, not just as exercises in pathological physiology?—like the last delivery I made. I remember it well.

Is that the moment I decided to try to become a psychiatrist? Because I thought I must tell my feelings to someone, someday, if I ever quit general practice. Maybe he can help me understand the little boy I plucked, raw and wet and red and screaming, from the bleeding episiotomy-lacerated vulva of his mother. And later while I sat there between his mother's legs in the glare of the delivery room lights sewing up the wound, I looked at the new life, now breathing quietly, naked and simple, huddled in a blanket. There was an independent being before my eyes, the very beginning of another extra-uterine existence. Yet I knew nothing more of why the earth had one more inhabitant after that last delivery than I did after my first, twenty years before as a medical student.

Again I had witnessed a woman's most profound biologic feat, her legs spread wide apart in the stirrups so that her fears and all her orifices were gaping. (How could I have been so curious about her anatomy at one time?) She had just shed herself of an eight-pound mass of squirming human muscle and a jelly-fishlike placenta. A few moments ago she had screamed in pain. Now she was lying panting and waiting while I sewed back the muscular walls of her vaginal vault, "nice and tight," as a male obstetrician smugly warned me once. "Daddy won't like it too loose."

And Daddy waited outside with a grin. Whether he liked it or not, he had to wear a grin and a big handshake. But I knew inside he was bursting with anguish because a condom broke and he shot his warm jelly inside his wife's sensual moving belly one hot night. She had some bad reactions to the pill. And now he had another baby to support by a business that was sinking. He wasn't sure that he'd be able to pay the rent on his hobby-store in a month or two, but he still had to keep smiling and passing out cigars while his guts were being torn to shreds inside his own groaning abdomen. So, both of them, husband and wife, with two little kids at home plus a new baby (he was all of twenty-eight, she twenty-five), had bad bellyaches that night. And I knew that their real problem was just beginning. But I said nothing to them, just smiled, and they smiled back.

So many other perplexities in medicine also constricted my coronaries and left my heart fibrillating with sorrow: A welfare case I saw years ago, a young black woman of thirty with severe head pain. She was dying: severe hypertension and renal failure. Her kidneys were gone. She whimpered, "Who's going to take care of my two kids?" She knew she was dying and nothing we could do would save her. Day after day her blood pressure remained high and no medication would make it stay down. I hated to go into her room and face her with the truth. I just couldn't bring myself to look in the eye of a dying person who knew she was dying. I felt helpless and so dammed mad at myself and at her and at God and at medicine.

I mentioned God. When I was six years old, my grandmother— who was always smiling and kissing me, who sang songs and baked chocolate cookies for me—unexpectedly died of a ruptured gall bladder. Nobody could explain to me why the doctor or even God couldn't save her. I could see they were only pretending about God, pretending even to themselves. I became a skeptic at age six.

I learned then that we are never secure or understood, not even in childhood. No one's pain is ever really heard by another, even when it's told to a psychoanalyst. Something gets lost in the translation. Are you listening, Doctor? I have you all to myself. Can you really hear me? I want to find out if I really want to become a psychiatrist and do what shrink-heads do and take all the snickering that goes along with being one. (A friend of mine who is one tells me that it marks him as a double Jew: once for being a Hebrew and once again for being a psychiatrist, the pariah among physicians.)

I know that even here I won't find out why that unwanted baby came to exist. Nor will I find out here why the black woman was ever born. I know only that she should have lived. Day after day she grew worse and her headaches became more severe, and I wondered who would take care of her two- and three-year-old babies, because even if their daddy cared, he worked as a truck driver and was away from his family for weeks at a time.

Finally she became dizzy, then nauseated, and her vomiting increased. Thank God (I don't know why I keep saying "Thank God"), she became confused. I was glad to see her obtunded because she no longer suffered the torment of fearing death. I knew she would never be lucid again, and I was relieved, and guilty that I was relieved, because my anguish over her torment was bothersome to me, and I wanted it to stop. And though I had wondered about that poor woman's black babies, I never troubled to find out because social service would "take care of all that."

Before she went, though, I wondered, why didn't the black woman break down and cry out loud like a baby? It was all over for her, and she knew it.

I cried once as an adult, but I stifled it. I was nineteen, an infantryman sloughing through the mud of Germany in World War II, scared to death of death. She failed to cry at all. Crying is a privilege reserved for those who have hope. When there is only despair, either you go on, for reasons I have yet to understand, or you fold up on the ground and give up and wait for death.

Unlike the black woman, I had hope, even in my worst hours, even during terrifying combat, except for the night when I was sure I was going to die. Then my omnipotence disappeared. Gone was the feeling that I would survive no matter how many others were killed. It was the night our squad sergeant strapped the gasoline tank of a flamethrower on my back and told me and my buddy to attack a German pill box. My partner, Wollman, held the hose and the nozzle. We had flipped to see who would have the gasoline strapped to his back. I lost. My platoon of about forty men was divided into twenty pairs of flamethrowers. We were to spearhead a surprise attack for the whole division, fifteen thousand men plus a battalion of tanks.

We were the leaders in a game of checkers, where the first few men are inevitably lost. Flamethrowers are easily detectable at night once they fire to burn up the first pill box. The Germans see the glare for miles and open up everything they have on them. The checkers out front are hit and burnt to death by their own gasoline. They're immediately replaced by the next pair of checkers, who shoot their burning gasoline and destroy another pill box and in turn are destroyed.

A few men have to launch every attack, and this night it was my platoon. I choked with fear. I wanted to run away or cry like a baby, or beg them to let me out of it because I knew I would be killed, but a man doesn't do that. So I didn't say a word, out loud. I cried inside without a sound or tears because I knew someone good inside of me listened and was more torn than I. So I could carry on, consoled by her anticipated grief. I knew she would never forget me for the rest of her life, even though I was just a heap of ashes, more than four thousand miles away in some field in Germany—my warm maternal introject who had always loved me.

What would people say at my funeral, I wondered (when the army sent my remains back home)? And in later years, would anyone (beside my grieving parents), even an old friend who attended the burial of my remains bring me back to life again in his mind, just for an instant, once in a while?

My heart pounded harder than it did two weeks before when we had to run through the German eighty-eight shells uphill for half an hour and then dig a foxhole in a hurry or be blown to pieces. I could feel it thumping in my chest as we sneaked forward in silent pairs. Each pair moved alone to try to surprise the huge concrete mounds while the whole "fuckin'" division—everything is "fuckin'" in the army—lay in wait behind us. I could see some of our infantrymen slinking noiselessly toward us a hundred yards behind, and I knew they would be walking over my incinerated body in a few minutes. Then the first suicide scout reported to us, and we checked out his report: We crawled inch by inch toward a small grating and looked inside. The pill boxes were empty!—abandoned the night before by the krauts who had pulled back to a new line. The concrete domes were silent, and it was unnecessary to fire a speck of flame. Again I cried to myself, this time with relief.

So why do some people cry? Because someone resides within them, an introject who says, "I care; I love you, and it pains me that you are troubled and that you cry." Those who are empty because their childhood was empty fail to cry, even silently. There's no one inside to listen.

The black woman had no warm black nanny inside of her. Instead a severe and rightfully embittered old woman resided there, an old woman who had been somebody's live-in maid most of her life. For thirty years she had been giving her earnings to help support six grandchildren.

In all ways the black woman was now alone. And the children would be left alone also—alone in the house to fend for themselves. There were no aunts and uncles, no family to gather in the hospital to weep for the empty life of the motherless little ones.

Her room was quiet when she died. A silent black man with a thin trim mustache and two little black children clinging to either side of his pant legs came on their bi-weekly visit. The children looked up at me so that their shiny dark eyes were accentuated by a rim of white. I told the father that she was gone, in words I had rehearsed. (I can't remember what they were.) I can only remember the two little ones, like a painting of black angels, peering up at me while the tears streamed down their faces; yet neither child made a sound. Their father had coached them not to cry. But I knew they had their mother inside of them.

In the weeks following the incident when I nearly became a heap of ashes, as I lay in a foxhole, I had plenty of time to think. That's when I decided that I would never return to the useless rot of my college days: literature, history, or philosophy. These were tripe: refuse which the army discarded in the dirt, expendable. Wasn't I lying there in slime?

But if I went into medicine, my knowledge and I would be cherished. I'd become the high priest, the most revered man in the community of mankind, the one who knows how to preserve life. From that moment on, any endeavor geared to anything but becoming the conservator of the existence of the chosen few counted for naught.

Medicine would teach me why we are born, why we are, why we grow sick, why we suffer, and how we can be cured. Shell wounds, shrapnel and bullet wounds, surgery, cancer, and heart disease, life and immortality would be within my realm now, and I would apply the skills of medicine to the only concept that really mattered—survival. That's what I learned in the war.

OK, you sons-of-bitches executive staff who spat on my knowledge and sensitivity and made nil of my scholarship. I'll play your game now and become an officer and a gentleman and rise above all of you in doing so. I'll no longer be a humble GI in the next slaughter or for the rest of my life. I'll learn more about your mortal being and how to maintain it than any of you, and someday you'll come crawling to me, the physician, begging me to save you from death. And by my skills and grace, I'll do so, smiling benignly, and you'll weep gratefully at my feet. I hear myself screaming right now. I still feel my anger.

So I made my decision for medicine as I lay sprawled on the cold mud somewhere in the valley of the shadow of death. I was deluded by the power of the physician, and I consoled myself with a promise for the future.

Then, lying in that same sorrowful soil, with the shells whistling in, another side of my ambivalence began to rise. I would not even need to be someone of significance, I begged, if fate or God would only allow me to live. To be the powerful physician? That was asking too much.

Again I prayed to the Lord Who I knew wasn't there. I swore to Him that if I returned home alive, all "the slings and arrows of outrageous fortune" would be merely blunt stones and wooden sticks buzzing noisomely about my face, and I would shoo them away with a good-natured wave even if they returned ten thousand times. Nothing would frighten me or trouble me as long as I could get up and walk and take a breath.

If a lifelong friend burned my house to ashes, scorched my soul, and stole the alms I had begged, if a woman I had loved for decades spurned me and laughingly shat in my face before my friends, if fortune kicked me in my tender scrotum till it grew swollen violet-blue as I lay helpless on the ground, all would be met with a resilient laugh and a hearty, silent, "fuck you."

I thanked the army for the philosophy behind those two precious words. Life would take on the sweet and simple taste of tranquility and nonchalance. Never again would I despair.

All I would need to do is remember the shellings one night over our foxholes in the German town of Geilenkirchen, near the border of Holland, and the screaming of Black and Godfrey and Heath when they were hit. No medic or any of us just a few yards away could get to them because of the exploding shrapnel. I saw one of them stand up momentarily and stretch out his hands toward us in his frightful struggle. Another of them kept crying for several minutes. By the time we got to them they had bled to death.

Those three from our squad of ten men, who worked and fought side by side for two years, and sixteen others from my company of 120, died that one night. It was the most dreadful sight I have ever seen.

Or I would only have to remember the mangled, silent GI stiffs lying on the ground by the dozens waiting for the big GM trucks to arrive, to be stacked like logs and carted off to graves registration.

And when my time to die came in my later years, I would have loved and been loved so fully by people whom I came to know intimately, and I would have known so nearly all of life's pleasures, that I would be ready for death and welcome it fearlessly. (Only a mortally fearful young man or a fool could have thought this at one time.)

But when I finally came home from the war, my indignant resentfulness at being discarded into the muck returned and so did my compulsion to become significant. I forgot my gratitude for merely being alive.

But one useful concept from those days remained—the obstinate steadfastness of crawling uphill under a fusillade of enemy mortars—despite my terror, to put my face close to the earth and to claw the dirt as hard as I could haul ass, with the mud and the sweat streaming into my mouth and nose and eyes, till I got to the top. I saw every other GI keep going, and I knew they were just as scared as I was. Once we got up there most of the krauts would be gone down the other side, or lying there waiting for us, dead.

I remember now something strange that happened on the summit of that hill. I still wonder: was it nature's way to reduce pressures, or was it the demand of our unconscious to reproduce, to replace those who were dead or soon to die?

For a few days we lay exhausted in the trench at the top. But when our exhaustion subsided, our tensions rose again, and so did our sexual urges! I thought of this also while I delivered that last baby: How surprising it was to me that within a few days of a bloody battle, I again began to dream of making love to a slender blonde woman.

One man caught Wollman with his right hand jiggling inside his trousers. The man yelled, "Hey. Look at him, banging away on himself, pounding his pudding! Don't you know that'll make you go crazy or become a fag?" And the rest roared with laughter and abuse at Wollman, the way kids did in those days when they had just been taught how dirty sexual intercourse was. I never believed it was nasty, except for some small part of me that warned that I might get killed at the front if I didn't wait a few weeks till I was twenty-one, before I sinned with a woman. My superego said masturbation was permissible, but vaginal play was for adult males only. During war, the God Whom I believed to be nonexistent meted out death if anyone angered Him even slightly. So I staved off my pleasures, and He traded me miracles like the empty pill boxes for my goodness.

My parents never condemned sex out of wedlock openly. (That's what it was called then.) It was their hushed silence which made me curious. I secretly read and re-read a dozen times the sex information books, with their pictures and drawings, that my aunt had hidden behind her bookcase, and I tried to peep across from my bedroom into the window of that good-looking Mrs. Zerost next door when she undressed.

When I reached my twenty-first birthday at the front, I was able to shed myself of that strange touch of guilt-laden fear. I felt that the Lord, if He were there, or fate, if it existed, would now allow me to have a woman because I had behaved till I reached majority and had not abused the ultimate of pleasures. Good boys were protected by fate. I found a dark, unwashed, starving, smelly, experienced Russian girl over twenty-one, whom we had freed from a labor camp, prison hovel that it was. I gave her all my cigarettes, soap, and spare rations to salve my conscience—even the chocolate bar I tried to keep hidden from myself for emergency use. Giggling, she sat on top of me on a chair, the only stick of furniture in her tiny room, and in her lubricious vaginal tract I finally became a man.

How disappointing it was to make love without a particle of affection or warmth. Still, after that I became driven, like all the other GIs, to grab whatever carnal pleasure I could in my race against death.

That strange force called sexual drive even drove some men to crime. One evening, a brown-skinned José trapped a little red-headed German widow in her farmhouse as we swept over the countryside. She had sneaked back at night to milk her three cows. Kumler, my Polish buddy, the man who once sadistically called me a "damned Jew," and I chanced upon them in the dark cow shed outside her home where José had found her alone.

With my own eyes I saw his massive body, still nearly fully clothed, lying on top of her, smothering her on the dung-filled wooden floor, her sodden dress lifted above her waist. There was a stale odor of old manure everywhere. He gripped her throat so tightly that her eyes bulged glassily from her pale, bloodless face. When he saw us, José withdrew, jumped to his feet, his fly still open, and stuffed his dark, dangling, semen-covered penis into his pants. He had hoped to do the deed in a moment or two and be gone before any of the rest of us might come across them. We called him a fool for risking his life and told him to be off. The payment for rape was the firing squad.

A few days later when a civilian government was established, she tried to press charges against him, speaking through an interpreter to the captain. When she pointed us out as witnesses, we lied. Kumler and I told the captain we saw them together, but no such thing as she alleged had occurred, and José escaped being brought to trial.

The red-headed woman's eyes were wide with rage as she glared at us in the captain's makeshift headquarters, her body quivering in a tense sweat. We perjured ourselves to protect José from the penalty of a momentary urge that could have ended in his execution. Death was too high a price for being a fool.

Do most men feel an impulse to rape? The boys and men with whom I was raised were steeped in a tradition of constant and sometimes deadly competition against each other (often to undo any doubts about our masculinity). At the same time we were subjected to guilt-laden, repressed sexual lust for girls. We grew up to be frustrated resentful men with fantasies of overpowering women. Finally our characters were melded in the fiery crucible of savage war. Can we escape the excitement of inflicted pain, the squealing, erotic torment of pleasure imposed upon a conquered, unwilling, and helpless female? In the midst of his attack, I realized: I, too, was José.

Some such as he even think it is a mark of distinction to produce bastards inside the bellies of their victims. I remembered that, too, when I delivered that last baby. (What has become of all the children who were conceived on a whim, an uncontrollable penetrating impulse, even a rapist's prickly surge?)

Does that libidinous seizure, the reproductive drive of mammalian man, undampened even by impending doom, that cataclysmic thrust alone explain in ludicrously simple terms why that baby was born?

Is there more meaning to life than a child's conception, a black women's demise, a war which forces existence to end for some and to begin for others?

I did learn more about that strange phenomenon called life when I returned home from the war to start college again; it became just another long and bitter siege. All the vows I had made became trodden and forgotten words, all, except that obstinate steadfastness.

The tedious hours of labor in pre-med courses, and the anxious uncertainty that my sweat would be in vain, made me unable to keep in mind one part of my ambivalent vow, my foxhole pledge that I would be thankful to dig trenches for the rest of my life if I remained alive. With the aid of desperation and chance again, I dug successfully—this time an array of fortunate grades—and was selected for medical school.

Once more, all my assertions that I would never again involve myself in an emotional mortal combat were totally buried with the GIs lying in the fields. Under extreme stress, I used my foxhole philosophy to tide me through new battlefields, for in medical school my fear of failure was as great as my fear of being killed had been.

Among the snipers in the wars of medical school was a professor of anatomy, a surgeon hot-shot who took pride in slaying medical students. "My job is to seek out the black sheep," he said, pacing about the room, heels clicking. He was assigned to the four students at my dissecting table in the anatomy lab. While we sat carving on dead Ernest (Ernest McQueen was the name of our cadaver), Dr. Neal carved on our table. He sprang surprise quizzes and grilled us on parts of the anatomy we hadn't finished studying yet, and each time he especially tore into poor Guilderman, bombarding him with questions that he couldn't answer. Guilderman was shattered, even when he knew the answers. Dr. Neal managed to dissect him just as surely as we dissected poor old Ernest.

"Draw a diagram of the brachial plexus," he pointed to Guilderman one day when we were on the upper extremities. This took place in a large anatomy lab used by the whole class of sixty-eight medical students with four or five instructors constantly circulating. No one but our table knew the tensions of this moment.

Guilderman, dark-faced and shaking, went to the small chalk-board near our table and carefully drew a perfect replica of the diagram from *Morris's Anatomy*. Guilderman had included even the minor nerves and vessels, which were superfluous, but he left out not one essential structure; then he waited breathlessly to receive his plaudits.

The other three of us were happy that Guilderman had scored a point. And damned if that thorny bastard, Neal, didn't reach up and with imperious strokes erase the diagram completely and demand that Guilderman draw it over. He wanted the diagram from

Cunningham's Anatomy because the trunks, divisions, cords, and branches were simplified in that book. The problem was that the class had been assigned to read *Morris's,* and none of us could draw the plexus to Neal's satisfaction. Once more he torpedoed Guilderman, who sank again, sick and faint. Only this time Guilderman didn't come up. Neal told the chairman of the department that Guilderman had performed abominably for the first six months of anatomy and should be flunked out at once. Instead, the chairman gave him one last chance. But by now, Guilderman was so intimidated that he shrank into a stammering, catatonic mess whenever he was quizzed. At the end of the year, the chairman of the department singled him out for a special oral exam, a grilling that covered all the minutiae of the year's work. Guilderman failed.

When the exam was over, we watched Guilderman leaving for home. He looked like a man who had been court-martialled and found guilty of high treason. He had fallen to pieces, weeping and angry, defeated, finished—unable to decide whether or not to kill himself, now that he had been condemned to the most sickening fate of all, the dreaded eternal self-damnation of a flunked medical school student. I heard of him a year or two later. He was still alive. He had decided to become a biology or zoology teacher, the graveyard of all failed medical school students and the mass of pre-meds.

We were left in sheer terror, the rest of the class of sixty-seven survivors. We shook and wailed and studied and prayed night and day, eating without leaving the lab. The stench of formalin sometimes caused us to vomit our undigested lunches of ham and soda pop. All the rest of us passed gross anatomy. Then the other bastard of the medical school, Dr. Hinder of biochemistry, put on his pressure.

Hinder was a Ph.D. known to wrench his ass to make medical students' lives miserable. He stammered over his lectures, stumbled over formulas, and made us all feel embarrassed for him when he showed himself to be unable to solve equations he wrote on the board, erasing them, he thought, before we could detect his errors. Yet his exams were exacting. He required precise answers to slippery questions on material that he took pains to be vague about.

Two more men taught the course with him. The first, "Rabbit" Twichell (called that because his nose twitched as he lectured), was the only good instructor in the department. The second, Moses Zurkeim, a disembalmed remnant from the days of the pharaohs, didn't lecture, but "aided" in the lab. Whom he ever "aided" was a mystery, but what were they going to do with a burnt-out, useless professor of biochemistry who never was any good to begin with and was too young to retire?

Hinder gave out his array of C's, D's, and F's on each exam. The son-of-a-bitch boasted that he had never given an A and rarely a B. His old exams were passed out and studied zealously by all of us. Collections were kept by frats, and he generously let us keep all exams to pass out to our successors. But he never repeated a question.

I studied, prayed, ate, and drank biochemistry. Even the daily few moments sitting on the toilet were not lost in mere excretion. Every moment counted. I read and reread his notes, swallowed as much of the book as I could, and entered into hours-long study marathons before exams. I prayed for a C, and a C was what I got, thank God, the grade that once was a degradation had become a salvation.

The sum of Hinder's final grades was twenty-eight D's, thirty-two C's, and seven F's. Each of the seven flunks was advised with feigned compassion by the creeping old bastard (I was told by a friend who received one and who is now an obstetrician): "It would be wisest if you dropped your plan to become a medical doctor since you show an incapacity to comprehend important biochemical concepts basic to human physiology." Guilderman had already been severed from school. The D's were placed on probation.

Imagine the old son-of-a-bitch telling seven men to drop out, just like that—men who had sweated out three to five years of premedical courses, the odds-heavily-against-them possibility of being accepted to a medical school, and the first tough year of medical school itself.

All of them had the right to go to summer school to repeat biochemistry one time. And five of them made it, passed with a C or better. Four of the remaining five were graduated. At the end of four years fifty-five of the original sixty-eight in our freshman class became M.D.'s. The rest failed except Teichert, who quit in bitterness. He grew disgusted at the thousand-and-one miseries heaped upon medical students, and he decided to go back into "pure" chemistry. Then we finally finished. The travail of years of premed, the ravaging concerns about getting into medical school, and the four exhausting years of medical school itself were past.

Our reward for graduation from medical school was a full week of vacation and the relief that our medical careers could no longer be extinguished by some disgruntled teacher who had been unable to get into medical school himself. Then began the grinding year of internship, a tradition of servitude in medicine, no doubt begun during the days of Maimonides' enslavement by the Egyptian pharaohs. We worked forever: sometimes twenty-four to thirty-six hours on, twelve hours off, seven days a week—five years of general practice and inhuman servitude rolled into one. And we saw pathology at the big County General Hospital that no doctor dreams of seeing in even twenty years of private practice.

After my internship I took another two years of general practice training: surgery, obstetrics and gynecology, general medicine, and then a dozen years of practice, and here I am, age forty-three, thinking of becoming a psychiatrist with three years of residency facing me, plus more years of training if I want to be an analyst too. I must be crazy! That's probably really why I'm here!

Doctor, what I've seen in medicine is a strange tale to be heard even by a psychiatrist: good medicine and surgery by doctors who care for patients and godforsaken tragic medicine and surgery by doctors who care mostly for themselves.

There was once a second Zeus, descended from Mount Olympus, a professor of internal medicine, Dr. Gordon Marvin, whose mind shone like a sun throughout the temples and hallways of the university hospital. He was the gem I once wanted to become. Even the children in the wards who continually cried or screamed, sensed his presence and fell silent when they saw him. Those who dared to look him full in the face for a moment could see that one cool grey-blue eye was a blind, fixed, immobile glass sphere. Years before he had developed tuberculosis of the retina following an autopsy. An ophthalmologist warned him that he would probably lose his remaining eye unless he retired. Dr. Marvin growled, "One eye is all I'll need." And with tireless energy he continued to scrutinize tissue under the microscope and drive himself to study late into every night. With only a small eye-spot left in his good eye, this cyclopian colossus saw more than any human being I have ever known.

When medical students made ward rounds with Gordon Marvin, a horde of sixty or eighty residents and interns trailed to listen to him. He made medicine a thinking game like chess: "What are the possibilities in this patient, in the order of likelihood?" he would ask with a squint in his seeing eye, a half-smile on his face. And: "Ninety percent of all diagnoses are made on the basis of history alone." He was right about that and whatever else he taught us.

I followed his ideas like an obsessed worshipper. When I was a fourth-year medical student, I swore by my stethoscope to try to become another Gordon Marvin. But my brain could not even begin to contain the enormous complexity of knowledge that whizzed through the synapses of his cortex. Does a patient ever know the difference anyway? Christ, let me tell you about one guy.

When I started my internship, I heard about the highly respected Dr. H. J. Visco. All the doctors and nurses on the staff of General Hospital agreed that he was an exceptionally good surgeon. What they didn't know is that he was also an exceptionally good operator. On my four months of surgery I scrubbed with him more than two dozen times—from hysterectomies to thyroidectomies, from chole-cystectomy to gastrectomy, from elbow to asshole. His anatomical knowledge and his technique were flawless. He even owned his own scrub nurse, "Bloody Mary," whom he brought everywhere with him, and she was queen of the operating room, commanding the interns on where to stand, how to hold a retractor, tie a suture, cut a knot, and avoid sneezing into the incision. She was Visco's exclusive property. Most other surgeons relied on the regular hospital scrub nurse. During his surgical procedures, Mary knew exactly what he wanted and when. Her efficiency helped his speed and skill immensely. Yet, when he shucked his wife of twenty-five years to marry another nurse, it wasn't "Bloody Mary." She was left holding his medical bag, weeping bitterly.

I tolerated Mary just to watch Visco's technique. Before beginning each procedure, after the patient had entered an anesthetized world, he glanced at the clock to pace himself like a good runner. He had a prescribed time allotment for every procedure, his surgical schedule was heavy, about three-quarters to one hour for a hysterectomy, one to one and one-half hours for a simple mastectomy, and so on. He was precise from start to finish, and he operated five to eight hours every day, then made ward rounds and had office hours. He had a fourteen-hour day and a cool half-million-dollar-a-year practice gross. He could have had more if he'd had room in his vaults, but they were clogged with cash.

By chance I was assigned to do presurgical examinations of some of his private patients. The university allotted several private beds for a few select surgeons who were on the clinical teaching staff.

One of his admissions was a woman with slight hypertension, questionably elevated basal metabolism, some increased deep-tendon reflexes throughout. In those days there were no thyroid iodine-uptake studies and no other lab studies to indicate hyperthy-roidism. He scheduled her for a complete thyroidectomy. I tried to talk with him about it to see if I had missed some of the findings that had led him to make a diagnosis of hyperthyroidism. At first he was willing to talk with me a few moments. When I mentioned my doubts, he grew quiet and looked at me as if I were an idiot. "How could an intern question the diagnosis of H. J. Visco?" his silence asked.

Unfortunately, private patients were off limits for teaching rounds if the surgeon so indicated, and this one was. He wanted no medical students, interns, or residents poking into his private charts—only the minimal hospital-required physical by a usually obsequious rubber-stamp intern.

So out came her thyroid the next morning. I diagnosed her as a chronically anxious person with hypertension, and nothing else. She needed her thyroid out as much as I need my penis resected because I piss slightly to the left of dead center. In the next few days I examined several more of his private patients—some, I agreed, in need of surgery.

Then one day I examined another of Dr. Visco's patients, a thirty-four-year-old woman with an attractive uterus. She already had two children so he might have figured that she no longer needed that offensive organ. It leaked menstrual blood once a month or so and was a useless burden in her abdomen. Objectively, other than persistent low back pain, which he attributed to her "chronically displaced and malfunctioning" uterus, there was no reason in the world to hysterectomize the young lady, not one area of suspicious cells in the cervix or corpus. Again I questioned him, not quite so innocently this time. There was "cause enough," he said. His face grew glum, and he walked away.

I noted that he sent very few of his private patients to General Hospital from that day on. He sent them all over to Doctors' Hospital and other private places that had no inquisitive interns or residents. I would run into him once in a while when I joined Doctors' Hospital years later. He still glanced the other way when we passed each other. I sent him not one case years later from my private practice, despite his continuing excellent reputation.

Then there was Willie Hamblin, another surgeon. Here was a man who wasn't in the same graft class with Visco. He lacked the title of clinical professor of surgery, nor did he teach at County General Hospital. The local veterinarian knew more about human surgery than he did. I would run into Willie at Doctors' Hospital and at Lakewood General, another private hospital that asks no questions of its physicians.

One morning Willie resected some poor devil's bowel for a ruptured diverticulum. By that evening, the man was doing poorly.

At about 7 P.M. he went into shock. Big Max Katz happened to be in the house when Willie screamed for help, and he grabbed Max to see the patient. Max had been chief surgical resident during my internship. He was a fine guy and a good surgeon. Willie had failed to tie off one of the big bleeders properly.

Max treated the patient for shock, took him back into surgery, found the error, and tied off the vessel, but the patient was too far gone and he died half an hour later. Willie informed the family, "The cause of death was peritonitis secondary to a perforated diverticulum," the disease that brought the man to surgery. Max just shook his head sadly when he confided to me that the abdomen was clean except for the massive hemorrhage, and the man would have lived with no trouble if Willie had known how to do a bowel resection.

Maybe you wonder if there was a postmorten? Even if there were, pathologists in private hospitals keep their mouths shut if they want to stay on the staff of the hospital that employs them. They might have thoughts, but they don't speak them out loud.

Nearly everyone on the staff knew Willie was incompetent, so he didn't have much surgery to do except on those patients who were unfortunate enough to stumble into his office by self-referral. Most of what he did was minor surgery, and maybe he got away with even some of the major stuff, but no one knows for sure how many patients were lost under his care. Only Big Max and I and the operating room personnel knew of this one. Other doctors on the staff of these little hospitals looked at us with horror when we mentioned Willie's name, but none of them said anything.

Visco was a crack surgeon without scruples and without prejudice. He continued to treat nearly everyone who came to his office equally. All were operated upon whether they needed it or not. He added two or three uteri a week to his surgical collection, plus various and sundry other parts of the human anatomy.

But Willie had his surgical privileges curtailed years later. Somebody on the surgical review board got after his knife. He could still do the "little stuff," but the executive committee of the Doctors' Hospital "requested" that he do surgery only with another qualified surgeon "assisting" him. The Viscos are never caught.

When I finished my residency, I decided to join a "clinic group" in private practice. The group said if I joined their twelve-man team, I would be an equal partner in a few years. Here was an established group willing to pay me a grand a month to start—big money to me when I was thirty. I jumped at the chance. Then I discovered that was an implicit yet well-defined attitude toward patients. Keep worried patients coming back weekly for a shot of B-12, or other vitamin shots, or medication. Everyone in medicine knows that, with a few exceptions, B-12 is explicit for pernicious anemia, not for "neuritis" or all the vague conditions of the central nervous system for which it's commonly used. Ninety-nine percent of all people given vitamin shots can swallow and absorb the stuff through the gut. If a patient wants a shot of this or that, "Give it to him. He'll only go elsewhere if you don't."

The practice of medicine was run like a competitive department store. Anyone with a cold got intramuscular penicillin, totally useless for a cold and dangerous because lots of patients build up sensitivity to penicillin. Any kid with a pair of tonsils needed them out automatically, though Lam, professor of pediatrics at my medical school, taught us this was balderdash. Only rarely do tonsils need to come out, when they are extremely enlarged or chronically abessed. Anyone with a bellyache that wasn't obviously due to eating too much watermelon had at least an emergency appendectomy. Patients with any kind of problem were instructed to come in regularly as long as they would come. Maybe one or two of the partners were more ethical than others, but their ambivalence must have been so great that they kept their protests to themselves. Also, by running a "nonprofit" hospital at a great profit, more cash was raked in. The dictum was money first, medicine second.

The wife of one of the founding partners was chief "nurse" in the clinic. The law has no formal requirements for a "nurse" in a doctor's office. Because she ran the clinic with the air of a commercial brothel, rumor had it that her only formal nurse's training consisted of working as a madam and tending those who fell ill from the clap and syphilis her girls passed out.

"Don't make a big *tsimmes* out of this patient," she whispered. "It's late and I got three more out in the waiting room." Or: "Isn't Mrs. Hangley's sore throat and cough pretty bad?" if I failed to indicate a need for another visit. Once one of the partners exploded while his stethoscope was still on a patient's chest and told her, "Shut up and keep your consultations to yourself." She screamed, "Bastard!" and never favored him again with her advice.

And now it suddenly occurs to me why her disdain for the authority of the doctor rankled me so. One of my unconscious compelling urges to become the doctor, even prior to my combat humiliation, my foxhole philosophy, my competitiveness, and my intense sexual curiosity, was that I had witnessed my mother's awe of the divine power of the physician, the giant who ruled over life and death, the man with the painful, sterile, steel needle and syringe—the great reverence and fear she had of him, the deity, and my father's silent respect, his quizzical expression, partially filled with gut-wrenching resentment at the startlingly expensive mysteries of the learned physician who came to treat my three-day fever and who was more skilled and respected than even the rabbi, and made ten times as much.

As a child I never dared to dream that I could become this man. I feared him too much. I could not identify with his Messianic power.

But in later years I mulled over my grandmother's death. The doctor's omnipotence, the infallibility I wished upon him, began to fade. Was he even a fraud? Ultimately, I dared to challenge the position of the king of men. I became Oedipus with insight. It was the army's "Fuck-you; who do you think you are?" attitude that allowed me to overcome the remains of my childlike trepidation even to bring to consciousness the overthrowing of the monarch: the physician; the father.

In medical school, aside from Dr. Gordon Marvin, professor and chairman of the department of medicine, I further discovered the doctor's mortality. And finally even "The Great Gordon" proved to have a great defect. He harbored a relentless compulsion to work and study in the hospital from dawn until midnight, seven days a week. He was driven by a desire to be able to astound his medical colleagues and students with the remarkable breadth of his knowledge. He sacrificed his personal life and his marriages to his cause. Everyone in the medical school was aware that Marvin, nearly blind, could see more and knew more than anyone else—more pathology than Osburne, professor of pathology; more biochemistry than Hinder, professor of biochemistry; more neurology than Russell, professor of neurology; more physiology than Siguro, professor of physiology; and far more general medicine than all of these men put together, though each man was chairman of his department.

A few years after I was graduated, I heard that his eye-spot began to fail because of further degenerative changes in his retina. Marvin became severely depressed. His obsession to learn, his only source of meaningful life, was threatened. The other professors of medicine agreed there was no organic cause for his depressive illness, only his impending blindness.

Two years after his illness began, Big Max and I visited the medical giant in a convalescent home just a few miles from the school and hospital where he had performed for over thirty years. He sat huddled in a corner, a bent, trembling, sightless human being, wringing his hands and repeatedly mumbling to the air, "I should die. I know I deserve to die. Please, please don't kill me!"

When he heard our voices, he remembered our names at once. He arose slowly and wobbled a step or two toward us, pleading, "Yes. Yes. Both of you are my students. Help me. Help me. Please don't kill me."

Then he became even more confused and sat down again, whispering to himself. He was preoccupied with his blindness, his delusion, and his fear of death, and no medical treatment, electroshock, or psychiatric care could reverse the depression of the King Lear of medicine. His knowledge and sagacity were beyond recovery.

I told him how I had respected and loved him as our teacher, but his mind was elsewhere. He remained in a corner of the room, immobile, except for the wringing of his hands. He turned his head away while he spoke gibberish to the walls. Then he pissed on the floor. His urine puddled around our shoes. I could see him lying on an autopsy table in a year or two. He was dead anyway.

So this is how a man totally dedicated to medicine lives and dies, I thought. His childless wife, his third and last, had left him long ago.

"The doctors who were once his students," a nurse said, "don't come to visit any longer. They've forgotten him." She looked at us with a reprimand in her eyes.

"Be careful of what is said in front of a patient," Dr. Marvin had warned. Ironically, it didn't matter much what was said in front of Dr. Marvin, the patient. And a lot his own staff cared about his cautioning anyway. Most of them, like Dr. D.V. Delbert, an arrogant surgical resident, seemed indifferent to the frightened patient who would have a dozen diagnoses thrown about by the "student doctor" examining him in front of a swarm of observers during grand rounds.

A few surgeons seemed particularly adept at terrorizing people who were nothing but clinic patients of a free county hospital. These surgeons felt elevated above the rest of humanity. They knew that clinic patients were placed on earth primarily for use as medical demonstrations.

Once I was assigned an elderly patient, a white-haired man, frail and thin, with an abdominal mass of undetermined origin. I was then on the surgical service, being quizzed by Dr. Delbert at the bedside of the patient. Delbert had me state all the possible causes of such a mass in an elderly male plus the poor prognoses in years of survival. Meanwhile he flashed through the X-rays, pointing out the suspicious shadows while the patient listened in pale silence. Then he cleverly read from memory the mortality figures to fit each diagnosis and left, snickering at his own cleverness, while the whole train of students moved on to the next patient.

I returned later to see my elderly patient. He turned out to be a retired Greek shoe repairman who spent his evenings reading Sophocles and listening to Mozart, and who had understood every word except for some of the complex medical language. Now for sure he knew he was doomed to die soon, probably of a primary cancer of the bowel with metastases widespread throughout his abdomen, including his liver. This was the first time he had heard his illness diagnosed, though he himself had suspected it.

A shimmering light behind his head reflected on the wall. Then it became a searing white glare breaking into dripping rivulets of diamond. He looked at me, seeming to have shriveled in the last few moments as a dead spider does after lying in the heat of the sun.

He said in a wispy yet gentle voice, "Even an elderly person wants to be informed of his death with dignity. What else does a dying old man have left?" Had I been in his place I would have wept like a baby. I choked back the sounds that came vomiting up my throat and silently cursed that fuckin' Delbert as if he himself were responsible for causing my patient's disease and all its anguish. I lied. Then I hated myself for lying, to protect myself, not the old man. I told him we weren't certain yet that it was cancer. He looked up at me and his face made me feel like a gutless fool. I promised him that I would never forget his words, and I squirmed out of his room.

I could see the white-haired gentleman (if anyone ever deserved that appellation, he did) lying on an autopsy table a few weeks, maybe a few months from then, same as I saw Dr. Marvin, stiff in the grotesque rigidity of death, totally naked in a final mockery upon human dignity. (Mind you, I have no shame about the naked ass.)

"An autopsy," I plead to his son and daughter, "is important for medicine. We help other patients by understanding your father's disease and the cause of his death." And: "If we discover any evidence of communicable or familial disease, it could be of great significance to you and your families."

I imagine I am doing the autopsy. The shoemaker's limbs fall limply in my hands. His cobbler's fingers, once dexterous menders of human soles, are now thickened nubbins, stiff and useless. His grey eyes are wide open and lackluster. His back is a violet-blue where the blood has settled in his new form. His front, face up, is pallid and starting to bloat. He stares and stares as if uncomprehending of the world into which he is entering, yet patiently, trustingly waits for me to begin. (He has forever now.) I hear the strains of Mozart's symphony in G minor, which he loved. Its melancholy fills the room and flushes into his vessels to dilute the acrid formaldehyde which has been injected into his veins. He and I both listen. We have this pleasure in common, even now. So he forgives me my mutilation of his remains.

I make the Y-shaped incision over his chest and abdomen (as I did during my training in general practice), stale blood running from beneath the knife in my gloved hands. I say to myself, "Did he know that his last involvement on earth would be like this?"

A pathology resident helps me dissect his remains on a cold steel table while people drop in and out of the room chatting.

"Did you see the football game Sunday?" asks a doctor who came in to observe the autopsy. "What a great pass Harris made for the last touchdown."

"Defense against anxiety," you're thinking? No. Most of the people in the autopsy room respect the dead not one microscope-full.

I hear the crude, indifferent laughter of the alcoholic aide who was an assistant to the pathologist. He was recruited from skid row, the way you recruit a sewer cleaner. He cuts out the twenty feet of bowel and with a water hose rinses it of its contents from stomach and rectum, the last enema and the last shit, and he cuts open the cranium to remove the brain. As the power saw whirrs on the skull, the room fills with a fine, sickening cranial sawdust that offends my nostrils and mouth. It is the smell and taste of a human being.

As I continue the autopsy and remove the organs, one by one, I, too, forget that just a few hours ago a man resided in this body. I feel like the butcher I watched as a child when I went with my mother to buy a chicken. First, he deftly cut its cackling throat, then proceeded with the evisceration. On the autopsy table, the patient's heart is neatly dissected, each valve examined, each organ, liver, spleen, and kidney cut, and slices for microscopic exam taken from each of them before they are replaced in a heap in the abdominal cavity.

Other autopsies stick in my memory also: The great, thick malignancies that grow in the walls of the stomach; the white-grey cancers of the lung that replace large areas of pink, spongy, normal tissue, the testicular tumor that metastasized so rapidly in a twenty-eight-year-old man (I can still picture the mass of tissue bulging in his brain), the leg I dissected from the body of a seventeen-year-old girl who died of bone cancer, her face thin and frail and even attractive as she lay before me, seemingly looking at me with an unhappy expression as if pleading to remain alive (the only pretty dead body I've ever seen), the dozens and dozens of "coronaries," sometimes five or six deep in the autopsy room, patiently waiting their turn to go on the table.

Death and autopsy with dignity, that's what I want, like the white-haired old man, because I can see myself stretched out on a steel table someday, too. If I can't discover the meaning of life, at least I demand respect in an even less meaningful death.

The first lecture we had in medical school was given by the professor of psychiatry, who pointed to the skeleton hanging in the anatomy room, saying, "What a noble end for a man—useful even in death."

"Nonsense," I said to myself. "It was just the sad remains of a life. How I would hate to hang on exhibit in public with medical students poring over my remnants, clanking my bones together and dancing a mock waltz with me when the professor was out of the room."

But maybe the professor was right. It is the last and most personal possession a body has to give away. I could say to my dearest friends, "Care to remember me by a few of my ribs, or a tibia, after I'm gone, or even the skull which housed my brain? I might look interesting on your mantlepiece."

My irreverent attitude brings me back to Dr. Delbert. When I gained the courage, I told him of the effects of our rounds on the white-haired man.

"Medical students should be selected more carefully," he mocked. "These days we graduate social proselyters instead of physicians."

I called him an arrogant, cruel bastard—to myself. I lacked the courage to tell him that hell was too good a place for his kind. I prayed that I could personally watch Delbert starve to death when he went into private practice, that no patients would come to him. I was scared shitless of him and every other resident or staff man above me, and I wondered where I'd gotten the temerity to say to him what I had said. He was one of those who graded me. My foxhole philosophy had always been selectively clever enough to keep me out of trouble. It protected me in the face of attack and shunned combat. So there I was, a quaking medical student fearing for my hide and wondering why I ever had opened my mouth to Delbert.

Reminds me that I'm like my poor old pop. He was a lowly Jew, scoffed at and spat upon as a kid by his German schoolmates. He, too, was always afraid of authority. He got out of Germany in 1939 one step ahead of the Nazis.

The German secret police had come to arrest his family, to pack them into trucks with other Jews to be sent to political prisoners' camp months before the extermination camps were operative. His father had been a professor of philosophy who was forced to resign his position at the University of Munich because he was a Jew. He then developed a mundane, yet thriving, factory that packaged custom-made dried and preserved fruit for gifts. My father and his family escaped death by bribing Nazi officials with a few coins of gold, which his father had buried years before in anticipation of such a fate.

His aunts and uncles and cousins who remained were never heard from again. He arrived on American soil with his parents, who died soon after. He was a pauper, newly become a peddler of vegetables and fruits. He settled in Chicago and remained preoccupied with the struggle for survival. He had little time for anything else. Upon my birth I became my mother's *goldeneh sohn*, her firstborn and only son and lover. She cherished me with a fervor that paled Jocasta's love of Oedipus and went far beyond her love for my father. I, too, was Oedipus (without incest).

My father had lived in a submissive-antisemitic state of terror since his childhood. When he came here and met my mother, a refugee from a Polish ghetto, they formed a jittery twosome, a *folie`a deux* of fears.

My mother protected me from all harm. She said, "Be careful. Do what the teacher says. Never talk back to anyone." I wasn't supposed to hear those bad boys call me a son-of-a-bitch. "Just walk away from them" Be quiet and be good, was her message, or we all could end up someday with our throats cut or in a gas chamber like Auschwitz.

It's becoming clearer to me now. I can see my past illuminated for a moment. When the people in the Polish ghettos faced starvation and humiliation, terror became her way of life. Her fears rooted in me.

My kind, protective mother's Polish-Jew anxiety, my father's boyhood lessons learned from the Nazis had gripped my impression-able childhood psyche. I also felt inside myself my father's humiliation as an unsuccessful peddler from Berlin. He earned a bare living selling canned fruits and vegetables to grocery stores on a weekly round, hauling them in a small truck. He termed himself a "wholesaler" to ennoble his work. When I was a kid, occasionally I went to work with him on weekends. Once I saw a grocer greet him with narrowed eyes and a flaunting, false smile. "Mr. Jew, I don't need any of your junk today." My father's reddened face turned down to stare at the floor for a moment. His forehead grew creaselined. He walked out of the store without saying a word. Was he thinking of the taunting Germans? I was too embarrassed to ask him.

I took on my father's passivity until an event occurred that awakened in me a startling self-discovery. When I was seven or eight, a neighborhood tyrant, tough and chunkier than I, sensing my cowardice, began a childhood reign of terror against me. He chased me for years, flinging rocks and rotten words and ridicule at me. I had darted away from his grasp dozens of times. I looked into the mirror at night and spat at myself for my cowardice.

One day when I was twelve, he started after me, screaming in banshee fashion, "Nigger-Jew look out," while his friends laughed. "Kill the motherfucker," they chanted. "Kill, kill, kill." I circled around the school in my flight and then in a preposterous, keystone-cop blunder, I ran full-speed into him in the school playground in front of everyone. I realized in the sickening moment of our collision that he never really wanted to catch me. He only wanted to make me flee from him like a terrified rabbit chased by a bullying hound. But we were exposed in front of his friends and he had me in his hands.

I fought for my life. I was my father seized by the SS. I grabbed my mortal enemy around the neck with every fiber of my strength, and I held his head in a strangle-hold, face down in the dirt, for what seemed like an hour. "He's choking to death," the boys yelled. "He's dying." I released him and he staggered away. Most of the kids cheered for me.

Through this corporeal, unintellectual accomplishment I recog-nized that there had been no need for me to flee for years like a soggy ghetto rat racing through the intrapsychic sewers of cowardliness. The U.S.A. was not my father's Germany. Gradually I emerged from my fearful, obedient, milksop stage into a cantankerous agnostic, challenging nearly everyone (except those like D.V. Delbert who awaken in me my childhood fear of being destroyed). In order to attain freedom from fear and a host of other needs, I strove for the supreme status of the doctor, who had control of people and events, health and disease, life and death.

Am I still trying to rectify the weakness and cowardice of my past, like wishing I hadn't fled from that tyrant all those years, or that I hadn't cringed before Delbert and instead had grabbed him by the throat, or that I had had the courage to tell that José had raped the farm woman? I live so many of the events of my life again and again in my thoughts and dreams as if rehearsing for the scenes in a play that has already been performed but whose ending can still be altered.

Am I coming to you to help me rewrite the script? My parents had been at the mercy of the world. Now I wanted to be the giver of mercy, not the recipient. I had been humiliated and threatened during my earlier life in the foxholes of my mind. There was no protection even for a darling son. No one could save my grandmother, nor would anyone shield me on the battlefields of life.

The morose and destructive Hinders, the sarcastic D.V. Delberts, the haughty Dr. Neals destroy people like Guilderman just as surely as the shells that fell upon us in the battlefields. And the exploitative Dr. Viscos mock them with Nixonish righteousness.

My parents' awe of the physician provided me with the delusion that if I entered medicine I would become the high priest of life itself and overcome the trepidation of my past and assure myself against the fearfulness of death. I would come to know my patients and they would come to know me. And I would learn what secret histories locked inside the skulls of my fellow human beings made them become what they are.

Yet after I delivered that last baby, I knew nothing more of life than I did before. Did I really believe that the brave and dying black woman suffered, or that the selfless shoemaker's pain was unbearable? Was my compassion for them only a compassion for myself, encased as I have been in my egocentric shell, wishing that my patients would love me as my mother had?

The Great Gordon ended in a rewardless tragedy. My father's subservience rankles me still.

So I have spilled the contents of my brain into your hands, Doctor Miller. Everything of my whole life, the cargo of my thoughts has been poured out. (Brain is only a soft, yellowish-white tissue, jellylike and malleable to the fingers of the hand holding it at autopsy. Be gentle with mine, please.)

Wait. A few drops still remain. To make my history complete, I must tell you of the latest part of my life. Time passed after my victorious childhood battle. The rest I have told you, except that I continued to grow and depart from my parents' ways. To demonstrate my continuing escape from them, unconsciously I sought for my wife a woman who was most unlike my mother in her fearful, frightened ways, and someone who would make me feel equal and better than the oppressor of my parents. Chance and time led me to an affectionate, lovely, virginal, broad-boned, blonde *shiksa* of Austrian-German birth, no less. Her family had a history, rare for a *Deutschlander,* of having opposed Nazism.

I told her of the oppression of my parents. She expressed compassion and warmth for them. This, coming from a girl of her descent, moved me deeply and made her irresistible. And she was shrewd enough to fend me off till she was certain of my love and special need for her.

Again, that eternal drive arose, that urge that has followed me, or more correctly (anatomically speaking, when I'm aroused), has preceded me (as an erection) all my life.

You said that you like to hear of every feeling of mine, Dr. Miller, and that one seemed to be there always.

Only on our wedding night did Lisa allow us to cling onto each other's bodies, till we melted into one, Jew and Gentile united, I to plunge into the deep and soft center of her warmth, rolling and plumbing deeper and deeper in rising, heaving motions of mutually convulsing international pleasure and tenderness. Then came the moment of quickening and inexplicable consummation, which established the acceptability of my family into the bosom of the people who once had expelled them. Then wilting and shrinking, I savored our love and my new-found status. Which reminds me again of the last delivery I made. I see that I may be as driven by my whims as any.

So I have seen something of life, dear doctor. I have become the physician, the one I deemed was the Almighty one. I thought that as a medical doctor I would learn the answer to how we came to be, and why we exist, and why we people are what we are. And all it did was make me feel even more troubled.

Have I confused you, Doctor, with this hodgepodge of associations this first day on your couch? Here I am the physician I dreamed of becoming, yet disappointed in being that physician; dissatisfied, yet ever more curious about myself; knowledgeable, but not omniscient; powerful, but not omnipotent; truculent, but not fearless; respected, but not universally loved, and still in conflict.

DR. MILLER: So, the first session tells the life history of the patient from the beginning to the present time.

Next time we continue to fill in the details of the past and also continue on what is happening inside of you this very moment.

How long will we go on? Till we are finished working together in this room. When will your analysis be completed? Never. As it should be.

Chapter 2
Further
Free Associations

The years have passed, Dear Intrapsychic Psychoanalyst. My analysis ended long ago. But it is, as you said, never done.

I come back to you again and again in my thoughts, where you began to dwell at our first meeting, between the living room of my ego and the attic of my superego, astride the cellar of my drives.

Then came the transference of my feelings onto you, and though it was to be resolved (which means you were to vacate when we finished), some part of you remains. I hear your voice, and I know you listen still to the journeys of my mind.

I tell you how my feelings are stirred by every patient who touches my consultation room door; often at night their silhouettes return into the reflections of my mind as multifaced moonbeamed ghosts.

I change from moment to moment and hour to hour; I alter from day to day as each person's tale unfolds and makes him part of me.

I am the patient who weeps for what might have been and who longs for the life that never was mine. I am the patient who is eternally angry at injustices done to me. I am the patient who travels forever in trepidation over illness and death. I am the patient who is never held in esteem to anyone's breast. I am the patient who dwells in claustrophobic closets of thought.

I am the patient whose adored child lies dying, and the one who has just given birth. I am the child-patient eager to please, confused by the world that surrounds me. I am the patient of advanced years who waits for the departed who never returns. I am the patient who lusts forever after someone else's wife. I am the patient of gloom who becomes the dancing maniacal soul. I am the patient of loneliness whose lover is lost, and the patient of exultation whose lover is found.

I am even the patient of reason and cheer, the one who can smile at the world.

I am each patient, one and all, and all I'll ever know. Listen as I tell you more of what has happened in my life since I left your couch.

Chapter 3
Emergency Room

How terribly strange! I felt it again—the same tension and excited, anguished curiosity and restlessness—my old sense of fateful resignation each time I walk into the cheerless grey concrete hospital through the somber, thick-metal, double-door entrance to the emergency room on a Saturday night. I've smelled the antiseptic odors and heard the quiet whimpers of pain in the air of the darkened hallways a hundred times before.

"There's nothing you'll miss in all of medicine if you spend enough time in the big county hospital," I heard an intern say to his fellow interns one night. I can still hear his voice echo in my ears. He was right. Everyone eventually ends up in an emergency room at least once in his life—sometime, somewhere, somehow—as a patient, or the relative or friend of a patient, or as a corpse.

The first auto accident victim I ever saw was brought into the emergency room while I was still a medical student. A seventeen-year-old boy had smashed his car into a concrete abutment at eighty miles per hour. I saw his mutilated muscle, raw and red, looking very much like uncooked beefsteak, his battered head and limbs, and the flow of his blood. He looked like some of the wounded men I had seen before on the battlefields of France and Germany. Later as an intern, I grew jaded by the endless procession of ripped and shredded bodies, and once more as a weary general practitioner, I was surfeited with the injured.

Now as a psychiatrist I attended from another point of view the terror and savagery of the emergencies of this vast, chaotic, and faceless city with its endless flurries of restless people and vehicles, moving, shifting, racing in the night, in the heart of darkness, in the immense loneliness of the megalopolis, surrounded by the huge sweep of roaring engines and the smells of exhaust, gasoline, and worn rubber that rose up from the fatal, blue-black shimmering concrete surface of the furious streets, until the day's choking smog finally settled. Then I drowsily awaited the end of the night, as the voices and laughter disappeared into the millions of cubicles that twinkle in the distant dark. The city finally was asleep except for the battle-wounded on the streets and the ill in their homes who were transported with sirened wings to the emergency room.

It was my duty, every tenth day, along with all my other work at the county hospital, to be the emergency room psychiatrist, one of the resident physicians, side-by-side with the surgical, general medical, obstetrical, and other residents who people this teeming hospital, this megalithic somber giant, grown enormous, swollen with the sick and dying of the massive city it serves. It was a psychiatrist's duty to be readily available to all other emergency room physicians, to circulate throughout the emergency room complex several times during his twelve-hour shift. In an urgent situation, he could also be summoned by the public address system to wherever he was needed. But even this small army was insufficient to quell the horror that awaited on Saturday night.

The emergency area of the hospital was divided into sixteen small, separate suites. I walked down the hall observing as some of the suites came alive. Every one contained four wheeled stretchers, one in each corner of the room, and a surgical table in the center. Aides and police continually pushed patients in and out of corridors on these stretchers. Other patients hobbled about everywhere in dressings and casts.

The doors of each suite were kept open as nurses, aides, and doctors moved in and out in a constant stream.

I stepped into the first emergency suite, where I saw a serious-faced intern named Dr. Hammond working at the surgical table, on which sat an elderly man gasping for breath, an oxygen mask clasped to his face by a nurse. The man, his lips and fingertips purple, great dark circles of black around his eyes, looked terrified. He felt death approaching. As he sucked in each breath, his shoulders and chest heaved rhythmically. Then the machine took over. The rhythm of the positive-pressure oxygenating machine made a hoarse, human-sounding groan, and yet, strangely, it also sounded like the oil pumps that moved continually throughout the California days and nights outside, silhouetted against the sky like silent, mysterious men of steel, bending and rising tirelessly, priming the bowels of the earth.

Oil was the old man's business. I had seen it written in the admission notes as I passed by. Now a machine similar to those that gave him livelihood gave him life.

Dr. Hammond reassured his patient with a friendly pat on the shoulder. When he saw me passing he called, "Abe, I got a patient on 5-C I would like to talk with you about if you get a chance later—an elderly gentleman who's confused at times. I can't tell whether it's functional or an acute brain syndrome."

"Sure," I said. "I'll be back."

He was a devoted young man. He approached every patient with warm concern.

In the same emergency suite, another man quietly lay on a cot. Curtains, partially drawn, divided this area from the rest of the room. Another intern, Dr. Mayburn, casually chewing gum, worked on the man nonchalantly, like a seamstress on a pillowcase.

"Hold still so I can get you done, Georgie-boy," Dr. Mayburn said to the black man lying under the white drapes, without looking up from the needle holder and the curved needle which he deftly, yet indifferently, turned through the sides of the lacerated tissue again and again, with a quick rotation of his wrist. He was sewing a long, deep diagonal gash that ran across the man's chest from his left nipple to his right hip. The holder rasped shut each time he prepared a new stroke, the gleaming needle slipping through to be quickly picked up once more as the needle holder rasped shut again and the needle was drawn out, a knot tied, cut, and a new stroke begun.

"Fifty-four, so far," the intern volunteered with a little chuckle, "and we're not even half finished."

"Dat's all right, doc. Take yo' time."

"How'd it happen, George?" the doctor asked matter-of-factly, still sewing. "I need it for my report."

"Is de police go git dat repo't? 'Cause if dey is, dey ain't notten happen. And jest between you and me, de boy who did it go be in heah befo' de night is gone. He'll have a real repo't to give you."

"Looks as if he cut you up real good, but you're lucky—nothing into the chest cavity," the doctor continued, inspecting his work with pride, while his jaws moved unceasingly on his gum except for pauses during which he held it between his even, ivory-white front teeth.

"You go see some a lot deeper befo' de night is troo."

Areas of dribbling and dried blood were wiped clean by the gauze held in the rubber-gloved hand of the intern.

"Ouch!" said George.

"Oh! Sorry, Georgie," said the intern. "The procaine must be wearing off." He plunged another syringe into the bottle, sucked up more of the anesthetic liquid and again injected the areas adjacent to the wound.

In another cubicle of the same suite the curtains were drawn shut tightly. Here a woman of only twenty-two, with a thin, slightly humped nose set in a long, pale oval face, lay nude between white sheets. Her abdomen was swollen full of life. Her bloodless lips were pursed tightly shut in muted expectation. Her long legs thrashed about, and she breathed heavily, looking exhausted even before her real labor had begun. Suddenly a visible muscular wave flowed across her belly. And just as suddenly her face, too, seemed caught up by a muscular contortion of sweated pain.

The intern had called the obstetrical resident, who tried to gauge his chances of getting her up to the third-floor obstetrics delivery room.

"No, we better deliver her here," he said.

Two nurses hustled for the emergency trays. The white-clad doctors donned masks and gloves and tried to clear the area of the people who occasionally wandered in from the waiting room.

A man clothed in a black overcoat and hat, a hand clasped over one eye, left the waiting room, invaded the double door of the emergency room, and walked up to the intern as he put on his gown outside the curtained area.

"Doc," he said in a low-pitched voice, "I've got something in my eye—I've been here an hour; I can't wait. I was walking across the street outside and something blew in. . . ."

The intern scarcely looked up at the man talking beside him as he went behind the partially open curtains again and wheeled the pregnant woman to the center area. Then he and a nurse helped her slide over onto the surgical table. Another nurse impatiently forced the man in the overcoat to leave.

Legs held apart by two quickly summoned male aides, the young woman, her pursed lips now parted, began to weep in a soft, pleading wail. The confused, hasty preparations for the delivery, combined with a hurried and embarrassing semipublic enema that filled the room with the odor of fecal gas, her relentless contractions, and her disappointed expectation of a painless delivery brought a tearful cry that was cut short by a knifelike pang that began in her low back, crossed her abdomen in a powerful sweep, crushed the breath from her, and threatened to burst her belly in an unbelievable explosion. It held for what seemed to her an interminable time. Feces spurted from her and spewed on the white sheets of the table.

The nurse mopped up, shaking her head. "We'll have a contaminated delivery," she said.

"Did you give her some Demerol and Scopalamine?" the resident asked curtly.

"A few minutes before you came," the intern replied.

"Hasn't slowed her down any!"

"Too late now, anyway," the intern said.

Another forceful contraction was accompanied by a terrible shriek, startling the whole emergency section into a moment of chilled silence.

"Take it easy, mother," the resident said testily, as if she had personally offended him by her untimeliness and her fears, and had no cause to be making such an uproar in his department. "Everything's under control. You're all right."

Another shriek followed.

The resident grew dark with anger, but he said nothing, only scowled at the intern for his clumsiness and for being inconvenienced, his professionalism embarrassed by the young mother-to-be. She should have waited for us to get her into the delivery room upstairs, his angry face said.

"Some night!" the intern muttered under his mask, sweat gathering on his brow, his hands shaking. He was torn between the irritated resident and the precipitating delivery.

George, under his blood-drenched drape next to the young woman, said, "She sho' must've had a powa'ful fuckin', didn't she?"

His intern, still sewing, unperturbed, agreed with an indulgent nod of his head and a slight smile. "One hundred and two stitches so far. Just a few more and you're off again back to your friends on Main Street," he said, disdainful laughter in his voice.

On the other side of the room, a third nurse said, "Have a few whiffs of this," bringing a small rubber mask down over the young mother's nose and mouth. The young woman winced and shut her eyes tightly; her face wrinkled into dozens of taut folds as the intern inserted the long needle of a syringe deeply into the muscles of her perineal region.

"She's going too fast for a first baby. Why the hell is she going so fast?" the resident said accusingly to the intern, still holding the intern responsible for nature's imprudence.

I longed to say, let the trembling fellow alone, idiot! Help him. Be less critical. You're only rattling him and causing him to be even more of a *klutz*. But I kept silent. The resident would have become even more annoyed if I had said anything. He was proud of his technique, which was being defiled by the younger physician. But why was he so callous toward the woman, who was undergoing the most agonized and traumatic night of her life?

The tremulous intern grunted as he struggled to conduct the delivery. The head of the infant—shiny, black, wet hair preceding—presented through the widely gaping vaginal orifice. A mixture of amniotic fluid and blood streamed from a beginning raw tear of the perineum, which bulged with the head of the child. Now the intern introduced a sterile scissors, incising the tissue of the thinned-out perineum to make more room for the delivery. A thin stream of blood was quickly staunched by the pressure of the infant's head as it slipped out.

"Wow!" said George, peering between the curtain from under his drapes. "Ah didn't know a cunt could open that wad'."

An indignant nurse, glaring, quickly pulled the curtains tighter.

"Now don't you tear anymore," the intern muttered half to himself, placing his hand on the infant's head to slow its emergence.

"She shouldn't have torn at all," the resident said, towering over the intern like an arrogant giant about to crush a gnat.

Then the shoulder of the infant slipped out as more fluid and a small amount of blood dribbled down to the floor around the makeshift bucket placed beneath the table, and in a moment, the remainder of the body of the infant emerged, moist and wrinkled, writhing and screaming as it clutched at the cold air.

All through this, a boy fifteen or sixteen years of age, with light blue eyes and a lightly freckled baby-face, sat nearly immobile on the third cot of the room, a large white dressing wrapped around and around his head like a turban. His bandages made him look like a huge, lethargic turtle with a Nordic face.

"X-rays look OK to me," his intern said. "I know it hurts a lot. We'll let you go after the X-rays dry out a bit and the X-ray doctor has a look. You can go back and wait in the waiting room and rest a bit, Tommy."

The dazed boy moved with a quiet whine, his eyes fixed in the vacuous gaze of a skull concussion victim. As he arose, he stumbled, slumping sideways. A small nurse with rimmed glasses and an unhappy, pinched look sprang forward and caught him. A male aide jumped up to help her. The boy clung to them as he moved toward the waiting room.

In the next emergency room a lump of a man lay on a stretcher, muttering to himself. He raised his voice and began to shout, then lowered his voice and again talked in garbled tones to some unseen person or thing. He was a vagabond of the night with a battered and pitted face, a few stained, widely separated, and broken teeth rotting in his mouth, tobacco-colored spittle dribbling down his unshaven face, a ruin of a man wearing a shapeless agglomeration of sodden rags steeped in the odor of stale wine and beer. He was a frequent visitor to these rooms, known to the aides who had worked here for years as "one of the boys" who occasionally stumbled and fell to the pavement on Mission or Main Street on any night, but especially on Saturday night when his working brothers from the alcoholic jungles of downtown were squandering their week's pay on themselves and any friends who cared to join.

Two husky orderlies entered and strapped him tightly to the cot with the efficiency of Gestapo agents preparing a victim.

"Hey! What's going on here?" the man shouted. "Let me off this bus; lemme go!"

"You've had a bad weekend," one of the orderlies said, buckling the heavy strap. "Doc ordered this for you—a little orange medicine. Here—drink!"

"Foo! I don't want any of that stuff the Doc ordered—just lemme go!"

"Up to the big ward you do go, you do go, you do go—up to the big ward you do go, my fair fellow," the other orderly chanted as they wheeled him down the corridor.

"Lemme go," shouted the man. "I ain't drunk. Lemme go!"

"Policeman said so," the orderly retorted. "Up to the big ward . . ."

The man began to thrash vigorously, throwing his arms into the air, striking the wall with his fist with a tremendous thud that reverberated throughout the room. His bruised knuckles began to bleed. The orderlies pounced on him with their knees, holding his arms as they tried to pour the liquid down his throat.

"Foo, pew! Paraldehyde," a passing nurse said knowingly, sniffing the air playfully. "Smells a mile away," she said as she sidestepped the stretcher on her way to help in the emergency room. She was a young nurse, skipping leisurely, seemingly on her way to a party, as she denied the pained and puzzling aspects of humankind that awaited her through the double doors she had just entered.

The first orderly, a wide-shouldered, strong, squat man, exclaimed bitterly to the other, "He should have given him a shot," as they fought to keep the struggling man from striking out again. They tightened the heavy belts around the alcoholic's waist, keeping him from rising once more. "I knew he'd never drink that stuff for us," the orderly continued breathlessly. "Wish we had a damned straitjacket on this guy. Those young doctors—they don't like to use 'em. So we have to fight these crocks like this!"

"The drunk tank in psycho is nearly filled already, and it's not even twelve," the other orderly said. He was bigger than the first but less malevolently muscular. "Must be a hundred of 'em upstairs already. Look out! Keep him down! Hey, take it easy, mister, you're all right." Again they shoved his arms down.

"Should've given him a shot, like I said, the God-damned intern!" the first said again as they neared the elevator. "Now look what we've got."

At that moment the second orderly, unaware that I had seen their tussle in the busy corridor, noticed me and cried out, "Dr. Sherwood, you're just in time. We need an order for this guy. He's fighting like a madman. He spit out most of the paraldehyde, and he's kicking like a mule! Can you give him a shot?"

A shot! A shot for this derelict of the night, to quiet him for his burly keepers, this hobo held in such contempt by even the crudest of mankind, these two handymen of human baggage! I've known aides who would have sensed the barren and hollow core of this squalid creature, but not these two! They were mere beasts attacking an emotional prey, barbaric in their ferocity, in their . . .

But wait! Hold! Why am I so outraged at the orderlies? Why such wrath at them? Is it because I am the real barbarian?—angry at their hatred, for it touches too close to my own?—angry at their rage because it reaches into my own bitterness, that part of me which holds disdain for some men, much as they do? Is some part of my own anger now removed from the alcoholic and righteously displaced upon his attackers, when I am his true adversary?—the sadistic part of me trapped into revealing itself?—my fear and anger and envy of my brother? Of a man who seemed powerful and free?

Yes, I had thought it was only indignation at the depraved of society when I was a medical student: how they brought their dirty, lice-ridden bodies into the crowded wards, overflowed the beds into the halls, inflicting upon me ceaseless days of unrewarding work, these nonproductive leeches of society. How many hours, weeks, and months I spent caring for them, resenting them, railing against them in some clandestine corner of me, against being deprived of my rest, or time to study and live, in order to serve them, these men who by their helpless plight required—nay, demanded—society to feed and salve them and labor fiercely for them, these distasteful, cadging vagrants, these grawing rodents of society, who foisted themselves on me, their leisure robbing me of mine.

Beneath this lay my unknown hidden envy of them, even while I hated them. And now I am ashamed of it. I have to tell the truth to myself, even though I had suspected it before in my deeper self. If I were unseeing, how could I expect two orderlies to know that this contemptible hulk, this tatterdemalion held clasped to the stretcher, is really Ishmael? Was he a child abandoned, of an alcoholic mother who was staggering drunk before noon, a painted prostitute on Main Street by dusk, whose father had forgotten him before his infancy had begun, his sire, himself a vagrant soldier of fortune, who tramped from bar to bar, from Baltimore to Los Angeles, from Hong Kong to Singapore, an itinerant sometimes-sailor, a ne'er-do-well who met a runaway seventeen-year-old dime-a-dance girl one night, fucked her and left her with child? Or was the bum destined by some cruel conspiracy of humankind and nature to be a foolish-minded, simple schizophrenic, or a mentally deficient manchild of whom no one knew or cared, or even the wandering scion of an upper-middle-class home who, for all the reasons contrived by wealth and "good family," grew to be this wretched, neglected mass of life, tissue, and brain?

And now it becomes all so clear: man's existence is merely the accidental interruption of eternity caused by the union of two cells. Born of pain, the screaming infant, with his first breath, sucks in the uncertitude of the delivery room, where, from the start, sterile masks isolate him from people and an incubator receives him in solitude.

How can I ask the aides to see what I, myself, have refused to see, to understand what I have willed not to understand? And now I know more of the truth, and I dislike this part of myself. My anger is changing into pain, but I'll say nothing—nothing except, "Yes, yes." Here's an order for the profligate. "Ask the nurse upstairs to give him a shot."

"Chlorpromazine," I jotted, "100 mgm., i.m."

The drunk began to flail his arms about once again, cursing fiercely, yellow vomitus and brown spittle welling forth from his foul-smelling mouth.

"Better wait," I said. "I'll give it now." I picked up a syringe, filled it, and plunged the needle, stabbed it into the bared gluteal region of my brother, my brother the bum, the derelict of the night.

And now I see the rest: from that deliverance the newborn child, struggling as if life is of some significance, receives respite for some long days, then enters into the agony of the aged, where organs, too old to go on, relent and surrender, and then helpless as the newborn again, and interrupted once more, the great complexity of cells, tissue, life, and work undone, disintegrates, fearful and frail, and alone again.

"My eye is killing me," the man in the hat and coat said, approaching another nurse in the waiting room. "I've been here over an hour."

"Sorry, we'll take you as soon as we can, but we're terribly busy tonight," the nurse said in a high-pitched, tense voice. She was one of the charge-nurses, a wiry, active little person who seemed to be everywhere at once. "Is this an industrial accident, a piece of steel in your eye?"

"No, I was just crossing the street and a piece of dust—I can't get it out—and . . ."

Two stretchers moved past him as they spoke, carrying people out. Then two new ones moved in, accompanied by the charge-nurse.

"It's a bad one," she said to the nonchalant intern who had been working on George. "A head-on collision under the bridge on the freeway. We have to move them in here. All the other rooms are filled."

The intern left George. He saw the shocked pallor of the teenage boy, then looked at his father and felt the father's abdomen.

"Should I phone to get the operating rooms ready for these two?" the charge-nurse asked in a strained voice.

"Only for one," the intern replied with finality, smacking on his gum. "One's all we'll be needing."

He straightened up, lifting his stethoscope from the chest of the boy. He shook his head, looking unperturbed, and continued to examine the father.

"Type and cross-match, and ask Dr. Randal to look at him. He's the surgical chief tonight, isn't he?"

The charge-nurse nodded and moved toward the phone.

A baby's wail filled the rooms. Its mother, behind the curtain of her cubicle, wept, relieved.

"He's a dear," the nurse assured the new mother—the nurse who had been indignant at George's peeping-Tomery. "Everything's all right, and your doctor's here now, too."

The young woman's private physician entered the curtained area. He was a dark-moustached, greying man, with a look of consternation, wearing street clothes and carrying a black bag. He stood awkwardly, looking at her, his now useless medical paraphernalia shifting in his hands.

"Came sooner than we expected. I didn't think so this morning when you phoned," he said. "First babies seldom surprise us this way."

I left the emergency room suite, just as another person, a small, frail wisp of a woman, entered the busy corridor. She wore an apron over her wrinkled cotton dress. She turned her head from side to side in bewilderment, her red hair strewn about a narrow face lined with patterns of wrinkles come too early for a woman barely middle-aged. There was a look of expectant horror in her small, dark, apologetic eyes, which shifted anxiously from corner to corner of the room.

"My son and husband are here," she said in a whisper, as if fearful to have her words heard. "Is it bad? The police called me at home—said to come right over."

"The doctors are with them now," a nurse replied. "They'll be out just as soon as they can. Please have a seat in the waiting room."

The red-haired woman took a few steps forward through the doors and swept the waiting room with her startled, unrestful gaze. I watched her through the glass windows at the top of the doors. A look of protest grew on her face, but the nurse walked off before she could turn around. The woman turned again toward the waiting room, stopped, and stared at the sign that read "Emergencies Only."

"I ain't never seen this part of a hospital before," she said to herself or to anyone who would listen. "Never even been in one before except to have my Andy."

One or two persons in the waiting room who seemed to have heard her nodded their heads, but said nothing. Everywhere, filling nearly all the wooden benches, people waited—fearful, awed, strangely silent as they hoped or prayed to themselves. Occasionally a few frightened whispers passed between family or friends while they stared expectantly at the fateful double doors.

A weary Negro woman sat in the first row, resting her head on her arm, her eyes closed. The imperturbable young nurse, skipping past, called out, "That you again, Maybelle? George back another time?"

"Yeah, thas' me. George is back another time!"

This was Maybelle, whose black, shiny cheeks had a cheerful orange glow beneath—Maybelle, who was known to many of the emergency personnel through George's frequent admissions, who tirelessly raised two white children by day and three black ones by night, the usually mirthful woman who cooked, and washed, and read stories to someone else's children who loved her, and whom in turn she learned to love. This was how Maybelle could keep her own family together—Maybelle, whose smile began to wane in recent days as she started to wonder after too many years of Saturday nights like this one if George was worth keeping, after all. He could never hold a steady job, and he didn't even want one. True, her children had a father, and he was a good man in some ways. He stayed with the children while she worked, even played with them when they were little, but then there were these nights, these Saturday nights when he met his old cronies, and they had a few drinks and began to carouse, gamble, get into trouble with someone else's woman, or quarrel and fight the boisterous rowdies who laughed and lolled the night hours away at the shabby, dim-lit little bars that line skid row on Main Street. How much more could she endure?

The husband of the red-haired woman was wheeled down the corridor toward the elevator, a bottle of saline held by the orderly dripped through a needle into his extended forearm. The nonchalant gum-chewing intern followed him into the elevator and up to the operating room.

A few moments later I saw the red-haired woman again, her face ashen and streaming with tears, sobbing violently, hoarsely, as she was led down the corridor from the waiting room back into the emergency suite where I was. She had been told. She insisted on coming back. She demanded it. The nurses had learned it was better to let them look. She saw a motionless body, totally covered, outlined under a white sheet.

"My only child!" she whispered to the nurse in a choked, throaty voice, her small hands clutched into two fists, her eyes alive with terrible disbelief. "My only child. It can't be. He was just home. He left with my husband just a little while ago. They went to the store to buy two bottles of milk for Sunday. They were coming right home. It can't be!" she said, groaning. "It just can't be!"

She shut her eyes tightly to blot out the reality of the moment, hoping desperately that she would awaken out of a nightmare, only to open her eyes again to the vision of a body silently lying on the cot before her, her son's blood-covered jacket and trousers piled on a nearby chair. She carefully pulled back the sheet, slowly lifted it from his face. Surprise and horror came to her eyes as she recognized him. It was her son. Still, she was unable to believe it, unable to accept what she saw. She nearly fell as she kneeled down to kiss the cheek of the boy they said was her son. Her tears overflowed onto his pallid, motionless face. Then she suddenly remembered.

"My husband. Where is he? . . . On his way to the operating room? . . . Oh no! . . . What happened? . . . Him too! Oh no! No! It can't be!" She said this as if she had never heard, although she had been told three or four times that he, too, had been seriously injured.

Throughout all this, on the other side of the suite, the tireless groan of the oxygen pump continued. The old oilman's eyes grew wider with terror and asphyxiation, as he became more and more cyanotic, a deep purple hue appearing over his face. His eyelids flickered and finally closed, despite his fervent attempt to hold them open, to hang on to life. The machine continued to fill his lungs with air, inflating and deflating with every other moaning beat.

I guessed that in his recent illness he had wondered, as an ill person might, how and where the end would come, and how it would feel, and now he knew. He was dying, and horrified, and totally helpless.

"He looks too bad to be moved to St. Mary's," the resident said on he phone to the old man's doctor. "Yes, we'll bring him upstairs as soon as we feel we can take him. . . . Sure, I'll tell him you're on your way here. . . . The family wants him in a private room? We don't have any private rooms here at the County. . . ."

The baby's wails filled the room again, as he and his mother, who now forced a frightened smile, were wheeled out past the resident on the phone. The white-trousered resident, sitting on the edge of a stretcher, leaned carelessly against the yellow-stained white wall, one leg wrapped over a chair as he spoke. He hung up the phone and said to his nurse in a brazen voice of arrogant self-assurance, "He's more worried about the family finding our hospital dirty than he is about his patient."

"Where mah doctor done gone?" George asked. "He said I'm nearly finished! Where he gone to?"

No one listened to George under the drapes.

The red-haired woman in the apron was back in the waiting room. Her sobbing continued.

"They were just home! They just left," she went on, pleading to the nurse in a mixture of incredulity and pitifully futile, hopeful expectation, as if her cries might reverse time, might resurrect her dead son.

She failed to see the covered stretcher pushed out of the emergency exit, rolling down the corridor past the elevators to the far end of the hallway. It stopped before the dark door of the morgue, which was silently opened by the first of the two burly orderlies. The orderlies went inside. I followed them down the corridor and into the morgue.

"Finally got that guy upstairs, Dr. Sherwood," the squat orderly said. "Hated to have to handle him like that, but he was really something mean. Here's what you need on this one." He handed the boy's chart to me along with the death certificate.

They removed the sheet from the dead boy's body, leaving him naked except for a cotton hospital gown. The boy had a thin mouth and nose set in a sad, narrow face much like his mother's, with a tinge of red to his hair slightly darker than hers. Then they slipped his body into a frozen refrigerator, his face close to the door as if pleading to leave, as they rudely locked him inside.

The squat orderly checked the tag around the boy's leg and neck. "'Andrew Mitchelin, age sixteen,'" he said. "Poor kid! His mother's back there in the waiting room takin' it real hard. In fact," he said, looking uneasily at me, then at the cold, yellow-tiled floor as if ashamed of his sorrow, his powerful square shoulders hunched meekly, "she looks to me like she's gonna have a breakdown, maybe. I guess you gotta talk with her, huh?"

"Yes," I nodded, "I've got to talk with her." And I left.

So the orderly who dealt so harshly with the bum really has compassion after all? Was I merely sounding my own feeling, a victim of my own rage earlier this evening, or could it be that the orderly had read my irritation at him and is responding to prove to me the better side of him?—the better side of all of us—his other face. Stirred by the death of the boy, the hateful orderly has become my brother. Like the bum, we are one. And so are the sick, the dying, the troubled, and the dead, the healing, and the healer, all one.

The redheaded mother—her son is dead! What is there I can say to her now? Let the damned surgical resident talk with her! He was the last to examine the boy. It's his job. Spare me. I want to deal with patients I can help, to bring health to the ill like the cardiologist, to bring new life like the obstetrician, to heal the wounded like the surgeon, not to be the bearer of death.

My anger was welling up in me, replacing my sense of helplessness and frustration.

I knew what she needed now. But where was the priest or rabbi, those procurers of words? I sell no words! I'm a physician, not a whore for a cleric.

I know we are all one—the healer, the soothsayer, and the priest. Let those bastards talk with her. Spare me the telling of it, the dreaded torment of the narration of death that freezes my heart and sets it to pounding with anguished pain and trepidation—the task of death.

My thoughts went back a few months to the parents of another patient.

"Mrs. Finley? Are you the mother of Alicia Finley, age eight?"

"Yes?"

My voice was tremulous as I grasped for time, stalling, hoping somehow she would know, hoping I could save myself from having to tell, save myself from seeing her face go through the explosion of surprise and retching horror, the sudden stab of grief and pain and resentment, and then her final rage—at me.

Mrs. Finley's face grew dark with poisoned expectation and knowing, her pupils dilating.

"How did it happen? How hurt is she?"

"A car—hit her. The driver told the police she ran out without warning."

She took a few steps toward the officer waiting outside.

"No," I stopped her. It wouldn't do to have them think she knew already.

"I—I—have very bad news for you, Mrs. Finley. Your daughter passed away, just now." And quickly I added, to drown out her reaction, "We did all we could—your child died just a few minutes after we got her—we did everything, everything possible."

Why do you look at me that way? Your eyes stab me with their grief? I told you of the death of your child, I'm not her murderer!

Why knife me with your stare? Why poison my soul with the fury of your wrath? Spare me the murder of my spirit! Your child was killed by another! I fought to save her.

My heart pounded with the anguish of the mother's startling, screaming pain.

I tried to save her! I would have done anything!

I reached out to touch the mother, to salve her grief, to share it with her, but her hands were cold stones. I was a stranger to her in a strange and frozen world, one in which her daughter no longer existed.

Where was my physician's mantle, my medical composure, the doctor who understands pain and fear, the immense, impending, eternal burden of grief that crushed her now, the overwhelming tide of emptiness and loneliness that suffocated her?

Another memory came back to me: A breathless, pale, middle-aged woman with a round, weary face and tired, puffy eyes entered. The emergency clerk had phoned her. The clerk had done as she usually does, contacted the nearest relative to say that the police ambulance had brought a patient into the emergency room of the General Hospital—no details on the phone except that there had been an accident or serious illness—cold, simple, and direct.

"Mrs. Kronowski? Mrs. Gregor Kronowski?" I shakily read from the police report.

"Your husband works at Ward's Clothing Store?"

I made certain there were no errors, dreading the possibility of telling the wrong person.

"Assistant manager, you say? Age fifty-six?"

She nodded her head.

"The police ambulance picked him up"—the words clung to my mouth—"about half an hour before you were phoned . . . Why so long? The ambulance takes a little time, and we were working on him while the police tried to phone you. . . . What's wrong? Please have a seat first. I'm afraid the news I have is very bad." A flash of heat swept over my face and body, my voice quavering even more.

"Mrs. Kronowski, we did our best. A customer at the store said he was talking with Mr. Kronowski and that he looked all right one moment and the next moment was clutching his chest, said he had a crushing pain, became sweaty and pale, and just fell over onto the floor. The ambulance came right away and gave him resuscitation and closed heart massage and then brought him in to us. They did all the right things, but by the time I saw him he was already gone."

"Gone?" she said, slowly opening her jaws wide, as if she were on a film moving in slow motion. The gold-filled ivory patchwork inside her pink mouth remained visible for a long time.

"Gone?" she repeated. Now her thick lips closed partially as the muscles of her jaws, bulging against her cheeks, tightened spontaneously.

Her face grew dark and hideous with grief and took on an ancient leathery look. She started to sob without sound, like someone retching before throwing up. Then she gasped, cried out, and vomited words.

"I knew it. I knew it. I knew he would die like this someday. They worked him so hard at that damned store. He had the whole place to worry about, the whole place, and he worried himself sick about it, day and night." She sobbed. "Sick—day and night. I knew he would die like this someday. I knew it. I just knew it."

She tried to go on, but a spasm of fierce sobbing strangled her and twisted her mouth to one side. A purple cast came over her brown cheeks. She gasped for breath.

Now my thoughts returned to the present. I was aware that the redheaded mother was in the emergency suite looking for me, her eyes and face wet with tears that she tried to soak up in a tiny, drenched handkerchief clutched in her hand.

Mrs. What's-her-name? Where's my slip? I'm still anxious, losing things.

I visualized the pale, thin-lipped face of her son lying in the morgue freezer, the curly hair of his head nearly touching the thick, insulated door, lying there waiting patiently for his mother, hoping she would visit with him, hoping she would take him home.

Here it is. Mrs. Helen Mitchelin. She was counting on me, praying for my miracle.

I knew that this "forgotten" moment, my talking with her, would last eternally in her memory. She would live with this night, and every word that was spoken to her, ten thousand times again. She would never forget the warmth or indifference that the universe felt for her on the night of the death of her only child.

I approached the emergency suite, still not knowing what I would say to her. When she saw my face, her sobbing stopped completely. She knew there was no miracle. Her gaze went through me now. She was out of touch with me and the world around her.

"I wish I could do something to help you, Mrs. Mitchelin," I said, but my words were hollow. They meant nothing to her. She was deaf to me, and completely silent. She just stared at the memory of her child.

The double doors of the emergency room swung open once again. The nurse admitted to one of the newly vacated stretchers a middle-aged, diamond-fingered man wearing an expensive dark brown camel-hair suit. He was doubled over, coughing, gasping, and wheezing. I remembered the sounds under the stethoscope, the squeaking, gurgling, moist rales. Was his the sound of heart failure with a myocardial infarct, or that of a severe asthmatic, I wondered? The intern would have to diagnose correctly in a few moments in order to save him.

The man was half carried by an aide and his skeleton of a wife, a shivering sliver of a woman wearing a mink jacket and a double-strand pearl necklace, probably a model, I guessed, half his age. Her blanched lips pursed tightly together in frozen fear.

"Put him over here," said the nurse, bending to help. She was the young nurse, still moving trippingly as she walked. She looked up only momentarily at the man in the black coat, who ran in again from the waiting room when the doors opened, one hand still clasping his eye, his other flailing his black hat in the air.

"Please wait outside," she said. Without looking up again at the angry cyclops, she broke her lithe dancing movement only for a moment as she labored over the new patient. "We'll be with you as soon as we can."

"Jesus! I've been waiting for over two hours, and I'm way late for supper," the man growled, turning his head to track the nurse with his good eye. "I've got something in my eye, and it's killing me, and what's more, I'm gonna catch hell from my wife."

The young nurse still paid no heed, propping up the head of her new patient with a pillow.

The man with the cinder in his eye stood alone in the middle of the room.

"Hey! Somebody's got to look at me. Hey! Somebody—somebody! . . ."

I left the emergency suite, left holding Mrs. Mitchelin's hand, leading her out, knowing that she needed someone still. I felt myself crying inside, united with her in our common grief, yet still isolated from each other. I knew that I would never see or hear from her again after tonight.

Working in the emergency room is one of the strangest and loneliest experiences in all of medicine.

Chapter 4
Belinda's Boyfriends

"But there is one strange guy I haven't told you about yet," she blurted during one of our earliest sessions. "This guy won't tell me if he cares for me, even if I say I love him very much. Then when he's no longer angry, he tells me I'm his whole life, that he sometimes feels that all he has ever done is really worthwhile because he's done it for me, that he thinks of me all day long while he's working, and that I'm the only one he's ever loved and blah, blah, blah, and so on," she said, squirming impatiently,

"Then in the middle of all this, out of the clear blue sky, he tells me he thinks of my sister sometimes, too! 'She's so pretty,' he says, and blah, blah, blah, and so on."

She brushed aside a few thin strands of long brown-blond hair. I could see her rapidly changing expressions profiled against the sunlit window beside her as she lay on the couch. Occasionally she threw her head and shoulders back as she turned toward me in an unconscious gesture of allurement. Her slightly rounded nose and clever brown eyes, made luminous by a quick, impish smile, betrayed in the transference to me her special status with him.

"How does that make you feel?" I asked.

"I used to hate him for it, but I never let on." Her thin-penciled eyebrows rose and fell, giving emphasis to her words. "I'd just let him rattle on and on.

"We've been so close for so many years, I've thought about our relationship for a long time. Finally last year I decided I would leave him, but he wouldn't let me go. I still wondered what it would be like, though. I finally tried it. I moved away to New Haven, went back to college, and finished my second year."

"How did it turn out?"

"Terrible. Every time something bothered me I called him. And every time I got lonely I called him, or he'd call me. We'd be on the phone for hours. Lucky he let me reverse the charges or I'd still be paying the phone bill. Then he'd yell, 'Look at my phone bill, sixty dollars in one month. You idiot, don't call me every minute.'

"Once he was sick and he tried to keep it from me. I could tell by his voice right away something was wrong. I begged him to tell me; I nearly went out of my mind. Heart attack? Something worse? My imagination never stops. I worried all night long. I couldn't sleep. Finally I called back at five o'clock in the morning and woke everybody up. They said he was better, but I knew they were lying. 'Tell me the truth,' I screamed. By now I was more hysterical than usual. Anything makes me go off that way, anything that doesn't go right!

"They finally told me. He was in the hospital. I nearly died. I began to scream on the phone. I cried. I peed in my pants. I would have fainted if I weren't scared to. 'Nothing serious—just some abdominal pain,' and they wanted to take X-rays. It turned out to be a kidney stone and they nearly operated on him. I flew right back to visit him in the hospital, and then I knew at the end of the semester I had to come back to him. I couldn't live without him.

"Now that I'm home, I see him nearly every day and I'm sick of him again. I love him but we can't stand each other." She laughed.

"If I don't see him for a day or two, 'Where were you yesterday? Who were you with? What did you do? Who else was there? And blah, blah, blah.' One night I let him have it. 'We're not married, are we?' 'No,' he says, 'thank God we're not!' 'Well, thank God is right!' And I slammed the door and left. He's not the only man on earth I like being with, you know!

"And I'm so mixed up—I can't make up my mind about anything! I like working with children, but I don't like teaching children. I'm a fairly good student, but I don't like studying. I'd rather be with people—and then I get sick of people and I want to be alone; and when I'm alone I can't stand it, and I want to be with people.

"And then sometimes my mind begins to race. I think about my girl friends. I wonder if Jean is out with Louis? He wants her to go to bed, but she's stalling—says she can't get a prescription for the Pill. And Gloria, she's been trying to go to bed with Mickey, but he's afraid she'll get pregnant, he says. She really thinks he's afraid because he can't get a hard-on.

"She bought him a dildoe rubber for a joke. Do you think he appreciated it! No! He blew up, then he started to cry. They've been going together for two years now, and he's afraid of sex. He thinks he loves her, but he's not sure, and he's driving her crazy 'cause she loves him, but he's not sure he's a he. He wants to try it with her and another man.

"If you ask me, she's crazier than I am." She slowly rubbed her soft, rounded chin with her knuckles.

"I wonder if Tom will ever call me again? And if Tom calls me, I wonder what this strange man I'm talking about will say if he finds out I'm dating Tom. I enjoyed going with Tom for a while, but then Tom began to bore me. Nearly every boy begins to bore me after a while. . . ."

"Does this strange guy begin to bore you too?" I asked.

"Oh, no—not really—our relationship is so much different from the rest—I mean he never really bores me, even when he drives me crazy. But then he's older and more mature. He's been around a lot, and I know he really cares. He says he's always loved me, that I'm 'the only one,' and I believe him. Yes," she said slowly, "I do believe him, because he is my father, you know." She laughed a little forced laugh. "Had you fooled for a while, didn't I?"

I smiled at her. "What does your mother say about all of this?"

"Oh, she lets him have his way—nothing she can do about it. He always does what he wants to do, anyway. My mother has always said to him, 'Let her alone—she'll be less mixed up that way.' But no, he can't do it. He lets my sister and my little cousin alone, even though they mean a lot to him too, but I'm the 'special one'—that's me!—the 'special one'—his first beautiful little girl and blah, blah, blah!"

When she moved, her large, full young breasts swayed sensuously, obviously unsupported by any underclothing. She half-turned to look at me, throwing her head and shoulders back.

"I wish you would tell me what to do," she pleaded. "You never talk to me, all you do is 'huh!' And 'And then what happened? How did you feel then?' Why don't you ever tell me anything? Tell me if I'm right or wrong!

"I'm not sure you really give a good Goddamn about me, really! If I didn't pay your bill you'd say 'goodbye—too bad—no pay—no lay—on your couch, I mean.

"I mean who needs this? At least tell me if I should date this new boy—he treated me awfully—tried fast to get 'smart'—said he'd have my pants down in no time! That sickens me! My dad would have a fit. Besides, isn't that all boys want of girls? Do you think I should go out with him again? Huh? Say something! Should I?

"Oh damn, I can't stand you. . . . You remind me of my . . . No, no you don't. . . . I mean you do. Well, you do and you don't. Oh God!"

Then I finally spoke. "So you want me to tell you what to do and be just like your father, don't you? Yet you complain that he always tells you what to do— tells you what to think and not to think. Seems as if part of you wants to mature and become independent and part of you likes the old solution best—'What does daddy want me to do or not to do? How can I please him most?'"

Her expression momentarily wrinkled into bewilderment. Her jaws remained slightly parted. After a pause she said, "I—I guess maybe that's right. You remind me of him in some ways. I talk and talk to him and he just reads his newspaper, and when I expect him to answer he says 'Huh? What did you say? I was listening, but I didn't hear what you said! Now you don't have to get mad just because I didn't hear you!' He makes me so mad! I don't think he's ever heard me in my life. I guess when you don't answer me, I think you're just like him, too—and I guess really that's my problem. He won't let me have my own mind, and when he does, I don't want him to. He wants to do my thinking for me. He says he wants . . ." She stopped.

"Yes?"

"He wants me to be on my own," she said slowly, "but he really doesn't, does he? Come to think of it, someone else said that to me a long time ago. Was it a girl friend? Or my aunt? I couldn't believe her, or maybe I didn't understand her, but now . . . but you know, I think I really don't want him to let me go, because I—I need him. I used to daydream we were married when I was a little girl, and now I almost feel sometimes as if he were my husband and not my father. Why, once when I was seven, when all the relatives were over for a family gathering, I put a ring on my finger, and I took his hand and pretended there was a wedding ceremony and we were married. They all roared with laughter and went along with it. My uncle performed the ceremony. And even before the wedding he wouldn't let go of me and I wouldn't let go of him. It's crazy, and I wouldn't believe it if it hadn't happened to me, like something you read in a psych book. But . . . my God, it's crazy!"

"Doctor, I've got to make a phone call. I know my time is nearly up, but my watch tells me I have a couple more minutes. Can I make the call?" She sat up, leaned forward and to her left, and rolled onto her feet.

Before I could answer, she went on to say, "I know it's unusual and maybe you think it's acting out, but it's important. Just before I came here, my mother phoned me and asked me if I could have supper with my dad tonight. I told her I didn't have time to talk to her and that I would call her back later."

She took a step or two, grabbed my phone, and dialed.

"Hello," she said. "Is that you, Mom? What were you telling me about going out to supper with Dad? ... No, I'm still at my doctor's. ... Why am I phoning from his office? Because I want him to hear. I've finally made up my mind, after all these years, to settle something. You asked me to go out to supper with Dad? Why? ... He asked you to call me? He's coming home from his business trip early, two days instead of three, and you're too tired? ...

"No, tell him no! Tell him I won't go out with married men any longer! ... You don't understand? Then tell him his real wife's not too tired, just too used to surrendering. ...

"No, I'm not crazy! ... What? You think my psychiatrist should see a psychiatrist? No, this is my idea, not his. Look, we're holding up my doctor; he's got other people too, you know—I'm not the only one! And I can't be worried about your husband and all the things that he worries about, and talks about, and blah, blah, blahs about for the rest of my life! That's your problem, starting now."

She looked up at me for a moment before she left.

As I got to know Belinda, I began to feel closer and warmer toward her, something I never allowed in myself much before, either in my personal life or in medicine. I could see what feelings her father was facing.

Her parents, like many others, had placed her in a tight bind and she was struggling to free herself, yet part of her was unwilling to let go, too, because of the unconscious gratification she got from their protection and from the intimacy with her father.

But then, how many loving parents really wish unambivalently for a beloved child to grow up, to become totally independent, and to break away forever?

I must stay aware of this in myself, aware of my relationship with my own daughter as she grows up, and even with my patients, particularly entertaining ones like you, Belinda, who become cherished, even "loved" child-surrogates. I've got to keep reminding myself to be aware of the feelings that are growing in me, too.

"The job of the analyst is to help his patients grow so they finally become free of him, too," that old geezer of a psychiatrist, and one of my psychoanalytic teachers, Dr. Barsi, used to say. And the stuffy old bastard was right.

Thus Belinda's analysis progressed from its inception. Her history and dynamics and her impact on me gradually unfolded.

"You said something to me last time, Doctor. After all these months of analysis you finally told me something about myself. I was so surprised to hear you talk so much, I nearly fell off the couch. I couldn't get over it. What was it you said?"

I uttered nothing for a while. I had said the same thing before. "You forget easily."

"Oh, it's coming back to me now. I remember—my father said something about my wanting you to be like him and tell me what to do and what to think. No, I remember all of it now."

"Still, I wonder why you forget what I've said so frequently, even just a day or so after I've last said it."

She replied rapidly. Her voice rose in a tense crescendo. "I always do that with everyone, 'cause I'm not sure I hear anyone right, I'm so mixed up. I can't be sure I heard you right." She laughed her nervous, involuntary laugh again. "Because my mother always tells me I'm the most mixed-up person she's ever seen. She thinks I'm crazy because I worry so much about everything and because I'm so unsure of myself.

"But you know, Dr. Sherwood, she makes me feel confused. She never lets me do anything without telling me how stupid I am, and how wrong I am, and how all mixed up I am, and why can't I be like my sister—she's three years younger—or even my kid cousin—he's only eight. He's over at our house all the time now. I guess my aunt's trying to give him away to us. Or why can't I even be as smart as the dog?

"Speaking of the dog, he's neurotic too. He jumps six feet in the air if the doorbell rings, barks as loud as he can, runs in circles like a whirlwind, and then hides under the sofa till he sees who's there. He's afraid of people, and other dogs, and even cats. He's a big, lumbering boxer, but he thinks he's a mouse. Did you ever see a dog that's scared of cats? Well, our dog is. He needs to come here too. I'll bring him next time."

She laughed again. "Who do you think makes me this way? Our house is the most mixed-up place I've ever seen and my mother is the most critical person I've ever known." Her voice rose even higher.

"She always tells my father to let me alone and not worry about me, but she still goes into her act anyway.

"Just last night she said to me, 'Belinda, look at your dress! It's wrinkled in back and it's too long in front. Whoever fixed that dress for you?'

"'You did, Mother, a couple of months ago.'

"'And why are you so nervous all the time?' she keeps yelling. 'From the moment you were born you were a nervous child. Even when you were an infant you cried all night, and nothing, nothing satisfied you. And you're still that way.'

"But then she admits how scared she was with her first baby—me. And because I was always screaming from the moment I woke up, she says, and something bothered me all the time, she didn't know when to pick me up or how to hold me, or bathe me, or handle me to get me to stop crying, and I'm still crying, she says. And she didn't know how to make the formula right to suit me, 'cause I spit up everything, or how to diaper me, or put me into bed at naptime. Outside of that everything was all right." She brushed another strand of hair away from her clear-skinned face.

"The doctor complained that she called him six times a day, more than any mother he'd ever known." Her voice became almost shrill.

"'Are you sure, Dr. Goodman, that she's all right? She just threw up. . . . What, try less milk and less glucose and more water? Why?. . . Is she allergic to milk? . . . What? Allergic to me? How could that be?'

"She couldn't catch on. And she said I was never satisfied as a kid growing up, always complaining and having temper tantrums. We fought all the time, my mother and I. God! Nothing was right between us. It still isn't. This is where I begin to cry," she said. The facial muscles surrounding her full-lipped mouth and her eyes rippled visibly as she struggled to keep from weeping.

"The other day we went to an engagement party for the daughter of my mother's best girl friend.

" 'How can you be such a schlemiel?' she said. 'You told Mildred that Daddy's business is terrible. You know you never tell people business isn't good, even if it isn't.'

"How am I supposed to know that even your mother's best friend isn't supposed to know that Daddy's stores are losing money? I started to cry, and I told her nothing I ever say is right.

"Women's clothing isn't so good lately and he's got a big overhead—rent for four stores and salaries for twenty-two working people—maybe because women aren't wearing brassieres any more.

No joke! Dad's places are known for their good boob-wear. He has a special manufacturer's arrangement for brassieres and pantyhose, and unless women start going bottomless as well as topless, business should be at least half-good after this recession is over, I keep telling him.

"Poor guy, he's worried sick, and so am I, but I don't say anything to him, not since I've learned in my analysis we need to let go of each other. I don't want him to know how worried I am, and he doesn't want me to know how worried he is, so we just worry alone and pretend the other one doesn't know. He has some money saved because we own our own house in Brentwood, ten rooms, free and clear, but still it's a big worry to think he might lose four big clothing stores in Southern California after twenty-eight years hard work in them—twenty-eight years!

"So on the way home from the engagement party my mother hits me with, 'How could you be so dumb? Nineteen years old and in college and you tell all those women your father is going bankrupt, and some of them are customers yet. Wait till he hears about this!'

"I didn't say that. I said, 'He's got business worries,' nothing else. So help me. But she lets me have it anyway. And when Dad got home, he had a fit.

"'I'm not anywhere near bankrupt,' he screams at me. 'We're making a good living, except that I'm losing my shirt, and I'll probably have to shut down all of the stores if business continues so rotten.'

"Then I really began to cry and my mother jumped in to point out that it's only a few months that business isn't so good and that it's happened before many times and everything's turned out all right. She says she knows everything will be OK but why did I open my big mouth anyway, and why, she says, did I wear that loud print dress, one of my favorites, when I should have worn the new yellow outfit from one of my dad's stores, the one that looks so good on me.

"Well, I wanted to save the yellow outfit for the next week's shower, and as usual, I started falling to pieces 'cause nothing I do is ever right, so I ran out of the house screaming, and my daddy was yelling, 'Where are you going, you idiot? Be careful. Don't drive if you're upset,' and my mother was yelling, 'Let her go; she'll be all right. I need some relief from that dumbbell,' and the dog was running in circles, barking from all the ruckus, and my sister was screeching at the top of her lungs, 'For God's sake, everyone in this house is crazy! Be quiet!' It was so noisy she couldn't listen to her phonograph records that were turned up so loud my head ached, and my little cousin was glued six inches from the TV, blaring away, and he didn't hear a word of what was going on. And that's the way my day went."

During one of our next few sessions, I had occasion to say, "So your parents tend to make grey things look black, and you listen to them, as any child would, and you see matters as dismal, desperate, and extreme."

"Yes, that's the way they are, and that's the way I am, and I hope I can change. Besides, I never realized how—'desperate,' you said?— 'dismal' and 'extreme' they were. Yes, that's the way I am—desperate and dismal. I'm beginning to see it now.

"But let me tell you, I can almost stand those desperate feelings if I have to—no, not really, come to think of it, but it's my social life that bothers me the most, that and my schoolwork—that's what really makes me jittery. I'm just falling apart, Dr. Sherwood, falling apart. And when nothing about my social life or school is bothering me, I'm all right, except that I'm always depressed and jumpy and I don't know why. So you see," she laughed again, half in self-deprecation and half in earnest, "other than that, there's nothing wrong with me."

I heard myself laughing, too. I was forced to join in her amusement at herself. She was always funny. Yet I knew how much pain lay beneath. Her stressed, rapid manner of speaking and moving, her appearance of being wound up like a coiled spring most of the time were her lifelong reactions to her parents. Humor was her shield.

"Also when I get tense," Belinda said, "I get diarrhea all the time. I get tied up in knots. Then everything shoots out of me. Dr. Hanson talked with you about that, didn't he?"

"Yes, he has," I said. I had discussed the psychosomatic component of her frequent bowel movements with the internist who had referred her to me. She had undergone a complete gastro-intestinal examination, including barium study X-rays, which revealed no organic defect.

"I'm embarrassed to talk about my B.M.'s, but I guess I have to. If I keep anything from you I'm just hurting myself.

"The other night I went out with a new boy. I was so nervous I couldn't stop talking. Talking is the way I deal with my nervousnesses—is there such a word? I just keep telling him about myself and how I feel and before I'm through most of the time the boy says, 'Gee! Have you got an inferiority complex!' It just pours out of me and I can't seem to stop myself. They all start out by saying how pretty I am, and I have no trouble getting boys to take me out, especially when I tell them that my hair is naturally blonde."

She took a quick breath and sighed, "So I'm very attractive, everyone tells me, but I can never believe them, especially if I feel fat and ugly, even if I do have a pretty face. Look at me; I'm sixteen pounds overweight, and I can't lose a thing. I weigh 136 pounds and I'm five feet six inches. I should weigh 120. My face gets bloated first and I look like Humpty-Dumpty.

"As a kid I was always a little overweight and the other kids teased me about it all the time. So I'd starve myself a few weeks. I just wouldn't eat and I'd get sick, but I'd lose weight. Then my mother would scream at me, 'You look like a scarecrow; gain some weight,' and my dad would yell, 'Quick, get her to the doctor's. Something's wrong with her.' And they just kept picking on me. And then I'd start to worry again about school or girl friends or in later years about boyfriends, and I'd start *noshing*. I'd eat everything in the refrigerator till my mother wondered if there was a plague of locusts in Brentwood, and I'd get twenty or thirty pounds overweight and bulge out of my skirts, and my mother would scream, 'Look how fat you are. You look like a cow. Can't you lose some weight?' And then I'd start crying, and the kids would start teasing me again."

She seemed to search for new evidence to explain her personality traits, now that she had built up some momentum. Her youthful forehead creased for a moment of triumph as she moved into a new thought. She sucked in her cheeks, making her full face seem narrow.

"But the worst part of growing up was yet to come. I didn't even know what it was to be a girl or a woman because my parents never talked about it, ever. They didn't even know if I had ever seen a boy naked when I was a little kid. My father hid from me, always slammed the bathroom door shut tight. I can remember that back to when I was five years old. I'm sure I never saw him naked once, not in my whole life. I'm sure of it. And they never told me the facts of life. They were so inhibited they never even said a word about the birds and the bees. They even blushed when someone mentioned that chickens lay eggs and bees made more than honey. That's how much I knew when I was almost a teenager.

"And one fine day when I was about eleven and I had just came home from school and had to go to the bathroom I pulled down my panties and saw a big blob of blood, and I was flabbergasted. I started to cry and I fell apart. I just fell apart. I thought I was bleeding to death. In those days the schools still were fighting with the parents about teaching sex.

"All I can remember is my mother blurting out that when you bled, you could 'start having babies,' and she raced into her room and brought back a book she bought for me to read for just this moment. But all I heard were the words about having babies. I threw the book back at her, and I ran next door crying to tell my girl friend about it 'cause I had no one else to talk to. My girl friend just giggled and choked and turned red and couldn't say anything either. It was all just terrible.

"The next day on the way home from school I saw my girl friend whispering and laughing to some other girls when she saw me coming. I started to run home, but one older boy,—he was thirteen or fourteen—must have overheard them. He ran after me and caught me alone, out of the sight of the others. He mocked me and said something about my having babies and then he grabbed me and kissed me on the lips. I was so surprised I froze. My legs refused to move one inch—first time a boy ever kissed me. Finally I ran into the house terrorized because I was sure that's how girls became pregnant.

"Kissing was sex to me, and now I was old enough to make babies. I was so scared I didn't tell anyone for three days. I just ate and ate, till I got up enough courage to tell my mother on Saturday morning, because I knew my favorite aunt, Cindy, was on her way over to pick up my little cousin. My mother burst into such laughter she coughed and farted. I thought she would blast herself to death. Now I know she was mostly embarrassed, not just laughing at me. I was never so humiliated in my life. Finally Aunt Cindy came, and my mother told her, and my aunt explained the whole thing to me. But I still didn't believe her or anybody else, and I just ate and ate till I gained thirty pounds in three months. Wasn't I a mess?

"Wait a minute. Now it's coming back to me. How could I ever have 'forgotten' this part of the incident? Now I remember why I really thought I was pregnant! That same boy, that repulsive, fat, ugly boy—I even remember his name now, Melvin Farmer—and I, just a week before, had been in our garage alone, and he asked me if I wanted to see his wiener. Like I said, I had never seen a boy's wiener before—not that I could remember, except maybe once on my baby cousin, or when my dog got excited, so I nodded my head. I was too scared to even talk.

"I knew my mother never dreamed that I could even think of such a thing, much less let a boy pull down his pants in front of me. So I looked, and I remember that ugly thing with all the hair around it, and he wanted me to pull down my panties so he could look too. I didn't want to but he pleaded with me, and then he tried to grab me. I was very frightened but I guess I was aroused, too. I made sure no one was around, and I quick pulled my panties down."

Her face reddened as she spoke. "He reached out and touched me up there with his thick fingers and suddenly I felt like vomiting. I pulled my panties up and ran out, and for days I felt sick to my stomach. I felt I was bad, terribly bad, and then when my menstrual periods began a few days later, I knew I was pregnant, not because Melvin kissed me, but because of what went on in the garage that day. Only I didn't tell my mother that part. With my parents there's no chance, no chance of ever talking something out with them, so I was just terrified. I couldn't tell anyone about the garage, not even my aunt. So instead I just went back to my old habit—my solace you called it once—and I ate and ate and ate till I grew into one large glob again.

"Isn't it amazing, Dr. Sherwood, that I remembered all that just now?—something I never thought of for half my lifetime, not since it happened. I'm even beginning to feel bad all over again right now just thinking about it." Tears came to her eyes. Her face flushed. She tried to force a smile.

"Now I finally know what repression really means. That's why I forget so easily. I'm such a hysteric. You're right. I do push thoughts right out of my mind because I don't want to think about them, or I don't really listen to something that's said to me because I don't want to think about it. I'm not really 'forgetting,' only pushing the memory away."

"Yes," I said, "I think you do understand what I mean by repression. I noticed that even your language and your intonation regressed to those of about an eleven-year-old as you were telling that incident about yourself. You sounded as if you again felt like the child you were describing. And part of you still feels like that eleven-year-old, helpless and fearful and condemnable. Your overeating was an attempt to allay anxiety by feeding yourself, as we've seen you do again and again...."

"But I'm not afraid of sex the way I was when I was only eleven," she interrupted. "Not anymore. My parents know I go out with anyone I want to now. They've even fixed me up with sons of friends of theirs. I've had sex-play since," she laughed quickly, moving her head and shoulders back to disguise her discomfort.

"Yes, but when you just described your life as a child, your affects and intonation were still those of a child. For a moment you showed us how you felt at eleven, by your reaction and mannerisms, by your response, your fear of criticism. You were the child you spoke of and part of you still remains that same child. It's that child we have to deal with right here and now."

"You're right," she blurted. "I really felt it—just like I did when I was eleven! You're right—my God, I really felt like it!" Then she began to speak more slowly. "I guess I need to learn that I'm really grown up, like you've said before—not to be like this child. But that's so hard to do, Dr. Sherwood, so hard, and I am embarrassed, a little, telling you all this because I do sound so childish. I've just got to keep it in mind, like you keep saying to me. I'm not that scared, frightened kid any more. But look at me; I'm shaking," she said, lifting up her hand to show me. "But I'll try to remember what we talked about and go over and over it again in my mind the way you said I should. . . ."

Belinda's sessions continued:

"It's when I'm with a boy I've just met and I like him that I feel so tongue-tied," she continued, "so instead of keeping quiet, I just blah and blah and blah. First of all, to start the night right, my dad gives the boy a cold stare when he comes to pick me up. Then my dad looks sullen, mumbles, 'Hello,' sits down, and starts reading his newspaper again, completely ignoring the boy. The boy just sits there squirming, not knowing what to say, and I feel like a jerk, so I say, 'Glad you two had such a lively talk. Well, I'm ready.' We both get up and say good-night to my parents.

"My mother tries to be polite and make conversation with me as we're leaving, like, 'Look at you! There's a run in your hose,' or 'Your lipstick is smeared all over your face.' She feels awkward with my dad just sitting there and she can't think of anything else to say, so she tries to be her usual self. I'd drop over if she ever said a few nice words to me. And my dad grunts something like, 'Goodbye,' without looking up. He'll never get up to shake hands with the boy. And we're off.

"And the boy already knows what a kooky family I've got. And if the boy dates me with another couple along and I don't know them, I feel like a sore thumb and then my stomach, I mean 'bowel'—that's what you doctors like to call it— tightens up and, first thing you know, I start going to the toilet again and again, and the guy starts thinking I'm loony 'cause I keep excusing myself ten times a night at a movie, or a friend's house, or wherever. It's that darn bowel movement feeling I get whenever I feel nervous. But when I get to the toilet I usually just sit there, except when I have diarrhea. Most of the time I don't even have to go, even though I felt like it a minute before.

"And if we double-date and I know the other couple, I still wonder what they think of me, and is my makeup all right and how does my dress look, and have I gained too much weight, and on and on and on. And then I start talking too much, especially about myself."

"And," I said, "you just keep talking too much and saying how bad you look to keep them from noticing it first and focusing on you."

"Huh? What do you mean?"

"If," I said, "you point out that you're overweight, or not too attractive, it takes the wind out of their sails. You just keep telling them how bad you look so they won't attack you first with that thought."

"You're right! How did you guess? Just last Saturday night I was on a date with a new boy and another couple. I said to them, "I'm eight pounds overweight, and my dress is so tight I'll bet I look like a sausage with clothes on, and . . ."

"So," I said, "you attack yourself constantly to keep from being attacked by others. Your parents have always been so critical that you now perceive everyone as being equally critical."

"Yes," she replied, "but then I'm critical, too. I not only have the feeling my mother and everyone else is critical, but in some ways I'm like that, too. I'm always finding fault with people, boys especially. My best friend Martha keeps telling me that.

"I can get along with most of my girl friends all right, but no boy ever seems to please me. If he's not good-looking or at least interesting, I don't even want to go out, and I have a rotten time with him if I do, and if he's not a college man, I don't want to talk with him, and if he's not Jewish, I'm scared of him, and I think he must be not too smart, because my dad says *goys* are seldom smart, and if he is Jewish he's usually very stuck-up or stuck on his mother, or too stiff, or too educated and bookish, and I'm scared I won't be able to talk with him because he'll know how dumb I am.

"So the other night I really got confused. The boy was half-Jewish. His father is and his mother isn't, and he was too good-looking and still he wasn't conceited. He has blue eyes and dark hair and he looks like a movie actor. He's studying prelaw and he said he enjoyed my company. And the best part is the worst part. He asked me to go out with him again. I'm scared to go another time with him because then he'll see what a mess I really am and—"

She interrupted herself, the anguished intensity on her face partially replaced by a smile.

"But I know what you're thinking, Dr. Sherwood. I've got to analyze what this means—why I see myself like that and where it comes from, and it's beginning to make sense to me, what you say. But it's so hard to change the feeling, even when I know about it. I keep trying to recognize that the feeling no longer belongs there. And it's true," she said vehemently. "I'm not a kid any longer. The feeling is from the past, like you say. When I remember it, I'm sometimes able to be a little different. I mean I really feel it, and I am different for a few minutes, but it's really so hard to stay different from what I've been my whole life, Dr. Sherwood, so hard, really! But I'm trying. You know I'm trying, and . . ."

She was working hard to become different. Gradually, steadily, her self-image was changing, but it took continued encouragement to help her put her new concept into action and to keep her from regressing. Yes, it was true. Her parents had stimulated and largely helped create her self-image by their own confusions and tensions and by their original interactions with her. Her father needed to possess her, and her mother needed to compete with her and to control her.

But Belinda had also to see her own role in the transaction: her identification with and even her exaggeration of her parents' attitudes, and her introjection of an even more hypercritical complex than that which she condemned in them. She was as hard and harder on herself and on her friends, especially the boys she dated, and more demanding of them than her parents were on her. My problem was to point this out to her continually, relentlessly in a nonjudgmental way that would be acceptable to her as she sweated to grind out new patterns of reactions. The danger lay in her seeing me as either of her ever-carping, demanding parents.

"You sound like my father, sometimes, and sometimes like my mother," she would say, laughing. "Yet I know what you say to me is so different. But whenever you start telling me about myself, I expect to hear their voices, except that now I'm listening better, and I don't hear them once you start saying something."

But then at times soon thereafter she again felt discouraged and troubled, whining and bitching at me again as the helpless-feeling little girl she often described to me so well.

How could I continually demonstrate to her that her reactions toward me in a myriad of different circumstances were similar to those that she had toward her parents, without unduly antagonizing her and causing her to shrink from her self-observation?

And how could I see to it that she was never permitted to get off the hook in analysis, no matter how vitriolic against me, or how cleverly amusing and entertaining she became? I knew that was part of her unconscious trap to usurp the very goals she wanted to attain.

I looked at her again. No, my droll, cunning little Belinda, you shall not take me in. You shall work, and work, and sweat, and work some more in our joint analysis of you till the day you grow up, whenever that will be, unless you run away from me and from yourself, as some do.

Time passed. Belinda continued her sessions regularly four times a week, through her second year, then into her third. Gradually the effect of her efforts began to appear.

"I know I'm less than perfect, Dr. Sherwood, but when I finally made up my mind to move out eight months ago, I moved out to stay," she said one day, "and I'm living on my own, no matter what. It's been hard, but I'm finally sure I can make it on my own.

"I have a cousin who is thirty-two who still lives with her mother, my Aunt Tillie. She's my mother's older sister—as bad as my mother, almost. Aunt Cindy is on my father's side, you know. This cousin never dates, and she's afraid to live alone. I don't think Aunt Tillie would let her live alone, even if she wanted to. Still, Aunt Tillie points to me as an example of what my cousin should be doing, 'cause I finally moved out. But unconsciously her parents keep doing to her what my parents did to me all my life. They tell her to be independent, but they won't let go of her. At the same time Aunt Tillie yells at her to look for her own apartment.

"I've been trying to get her to a psychiatrist for years, but they won't let her go, especially after they've seen what happened to me. Poor kid! She's an only child, and they just don't want to lose their baby.

"One day I told Aunt Tillie if it weren't for my analysis I'd still be living at home, the same sick person I was three years ago. Aunt Tillie listened, and marveled, and I thought she was going to scream, 'Quick, give me your psychiatrist's name.' But she didn't, and she still hasn't taken my cousin to anyone, especially not during these past few months, because my mother has been telling her how much I've been letting her have it lately.

"So Aunt Tillie's gotten even more scared of psychiatry." Her laughter rose again. "She doesn't want her daughter to be that well.

"Now when my mother comes over, I just don't take any more crap from her. That's right." She smiled. "No more crap. You've always been telling me how hard I am on myself and how I criticize myself the way my mother does and how hysterical I am. I'm really looking at myself all the time now. School's killing me, but I've only got this one semester left and then I'll go out and try to get a job teaching. Then I won't need any more money from them, and I'll really be on my own. I can't believe it. I've been living on my own for more than half a year. I never thought I could, and neither did my mother. I'm sorry to disappoint her.

"The other night she and my dad came over, and she was looking for trouble again. She began to say something about the way my apartment was a complete mess, and that my kitchen was smelly from old food stuck on the table and counters, and the refrigerator needed cleaning and straightening, and my filthy laundry was piling up, and my yellow curtains were dirty and wrinkled, and she would've gone on and on for an hour if I hadn't stopped her and said, 'Be quiet! This is my apartment, and you're a guest, so be quiet and enjoy what I give you for supper.' She couldn't believe her ears. She started choking and coughing over the spaghetti and meat balls I made for them, like she does whenever she's upset, but this time I meant what I said, and she knew it.

"She's not used to the new me, and every time I start talking like that she hints about stopping paying for my analysis. Then my dad pipes up and says, 'Analysis is doing Belinda a world of good,' and he just gives her a dirty look.

"That's until I say something he doesn't like, and then he threatens to cut out my analysis, and she says, 'Look how our baby's grown up in the last couple of years. She sounds like a woman now. Let her alone! If you won't pay for it, I will.' Then they both begin to fight like a couple of cackling mad hens until I finally tell them, 'For God's sake! as soon as I get a job I'll pay for my own God-damned analysis,' and that shuts them both up."

After a few more months of our work, she said to me, "Psychoanalysis has really been good for me. It's still killing me, but it's been good for me," she laughed, throwing her shoulders back. "You won't let me get away with anything. I used to kid myself and say I couldn't do it—finish school, or live away from home, or make almost any decision for myself, but you urged me to think of taking a chance." She laughed. "And just look what progress I've made! Just look at me. I'm a wreck! A mess! I've lost all the weight I need to just worrying about taking care of myself. So here I am, more independent and free, but all wrinkled and shriveled up like a woman of sixty. No kidding! I saw wrinkles this morning when I looked in the mirror—from worrying about taking care of myself this last year. Psychiatry is doing me a lot of good, making me look old—old at twenty-two." She smiled.

"Still, I'm doing things I never dreamed I could do before, like mingling with all the young people every day in this huge apartment I'm in. But best of all," her brown eyes shone, "this guy who is so good-looking is after me again. You remember, Robert, the one I told you about who's a half-breed—half-Jew, half-goy. I dated him once or twice a long time ago. Well, he went away to the service and I didn't hear from him for almost two years. And now, out of nowhere, he called me again and said he's back and wanted to see me, and I've dated him three times this week already." She swallowed quickly. "And I think I'm in love—terribly in love with him. I'm not nearly as critical of Robert as I usually am of boys. I can stand some of his faults, or what I used to think were faults in boys, like being too short, or having B.O., or having a kooky family, or not having much money, or not being well established in a business or a career. I think I've grown up from all these years of looking at how demanding I've been of guys and of everyone else, including myself.

"Now if the seam of my dress isn't exactly as straight as it should be, or if it's a little too tight over my ass 'cause I'm a few pounds overweight, or if my stockings don't exactly match my outfit, or if one of my girl friends thinks I said something stupid on a double date, I don't give a damn. Or at least I don't care so much that it worries me to death the way it used to. I've finally decided that no one thinks about me nearly as much as I think they do ..."

A few months later Belinda entered, talking briskly as she moved toward the couch. "You think I've had problems till now, Dr. Sherwood? Believe me. Now I've really got problems! Robert and I were arguing all night long about my moving into his apartment with him, or having him move into mine, and I want to do it, but—but why not, damn it? It's what I want and he wants, and fuck my mother and dad! That's right, fuck them. And you, too. You heard me right the first time. You look so shocked." She grinned. "Your mouth is hanging open."

"Not quite shocked," I said. "Just surprised. You sound as if—"

"As if I know what I want to do and I'm going to do it, no matter what you or anyone else says." She looked at me directly, turning her head around on the couch in order to view me fully. There was an expectation of disapproval from me in her expression.

"You know I've been going with him all these months, and I told you how I began to feel about Robert. He feels that way about me, too. We're in love. We fight like a couple of scrapping alley cats, but we love each other. That reminds me of what my mother said to me a year or two ago about boys when she heard that I even knew a non-Jewish boy. 'I don't care whom you marry. Marry anyone you want. Just remember if he's not Jewish, your father will kill himself, so just take your time and pick out the right *shaygets.*'

"Well, Robert ought to be at least half acceptable to my parents 'cause he's half Jewish. Such prejudice! I wouldn't care if he were half Arab, if I loved him."

She paused, thoughtful. "I'm glad we've been able to talk so openly about sex in here. Because I finally tried it with him." Her face, now nearly free of acne, flushed faintly as she spoke, a half-determined look replacing an embarrassed smile. After all these years of thinking sex would be horrible after what happened to me as a kid with Melvin and all and my parents' attitudes, it was great—for him! She laughed. "For me it was great, too, a great big flop! I can begin to enjoy it when we're petting—" she broke off.

"It's amazing I can talk about it this way. I never believed I'd be able to before, but working on these feelings about it all this time did help me. I wasn't revolted the way I thought I'd be. One of the few things my mother ever told me about sex is that she vomited the first time she tried it with my dad—actually vomited." She chuckled. "How's that for a wholesome lecture on sex education? She just told me about it a few weeks ago, probably to scare me, because she was getting suspicious about Robert and me. But that's actually her attitude—the one she tried to give me all of her life—that sex is some dirty thing you shouldn't think about if you're a nice girl ..."

A few weeks later, Belinda looked down at the floor as she walked across the room to the couch, avoiding my eyes.

"This business of orgasm, Dr. Sherwood, it bothers me," she began. "Everyone says it's so important and I can't seem to have one, no matter how hard I try. He's tried to encourage me, but nothing seems to help.

"If my mother heard me talking now she'd drop dead. She wouldn't believe her ears to hear anyone, especially her little girl, talking this way to someone, even a medical doctor.

"Anyway, what about that thing called orgasm? I've heard some girl friends talk about it, and I've read about it in books like Masters and Johnson, but it still doesn't help. I do have to admit," she paused, her face reddening again, "that I'm not really as comfortable with the whole damned thing as I sound, 'cause I'm actually scared stiff of the whole thing, of the stiff itself." She giggled. 'I'm really not at ease when we try anything. I feel terrible, as if I'm sneaking around doing something dirty. In fact," she went on, her voice dropping, "it even hurts like hell sometimes, but I just put up with it because I'm supposed to, and I don't want Robert to think I'm not having lots of pleasure, the way the sensuous female should."

Her face, bursting with the humiliation she was concealing from even herself, suddenly reddened and spilled forth the stream of tears she had tried to suppress. "I finally find somebody I care for and we're having a miserable time. And it's not just sex I'm talking about. He thinks I'm too up-tight about everything. He's constantly yelling at me to relax and not to worry so much about my school work or anything else."

She wiped her nose with a soggy tissue. "That's easy for him to say until he starts talking about his own courses. Then you should hear how he starts whining and swearing about the God-damned A he just missed in Business Math 203 or the C some senile creep gave him in an important prelaw course.

" 'Exams are coming up,' he says. 'I won't be able to see you this weekend, and besides, you're not much fun anymore. I'm going back to my own apartment for now.'

"Well, how can I keep from worrying when he says I don't know how to make love. He compares me with some of the other girls he's gone to bed with, including one girl he used to live with, a slut he picked up in a bar. So now that I'm not worrying much about all the little things I used to worry about my whole life, I've got something real to worry about. Lucky me! And when he drinks a lot he starts getting mean and yelling things like, 'You're like a sack of potatoes in bed, you fuckin' Jewish princess.'

"I remind him that he didn't meet me while I was dead drunk at some dingy saloon where the beach bums hang out, and that I'm not very experienced at being a whore, like his good old Agnes. I'm just not going to chase him everywhere he goes, the way all his other girl friends did, and be his mistress, on call day and night. I told him that—more than once. And when I do, he pouts like a spoiled little boy, runs off to his favorite drinking place again, and comes back to my apartment stoned and drunk.

"Then he's really mean! That's how I found out his mother committed suicide. A few weeks ago he stumbled into my apartment so drunk he could hardly walk. We started living together, you know. But that night he became somebody else, not the boy I was living with, just somebody I never knew.

"The muscles of her face tightened, causing her jaw to jut forward defiantly. "He looked mean, and he frightened the hell out of me. He called me a 'dirty cunt,' and he grabbed my arm and twisted it hard, and threw me down, and he was going to hit me in the face with his fist, the way he used to beat up on Agnes when he was drunk."

She seemed to stop breathing. "I was never so scared in my life! Something inside of me made me scream at him that I just wasn't any girl he had dragged in off the street, that he'd said he loved me, or I wouldn't be living with him. He let go of me, and turned pale, and walked away. I couldn't believe it. It all seemed like some frightening second-rate TV movie. But it was true.

"His mother left him, he said, when he was only four or five. He says she 'left,' because that's what he was told by his father just after his parents were divorced. Robert was living alone with his mother, but one day he came home from nursery school in a car pool and found his father there. His dad was a bank official, pretty well-to-do, and he told Robert that his mother just went far away and that he would never see her again, and that he would have to live with an aunt whom Robert never did like. His father couldn't keep him or didn't want to.

"Poor Robert was confused and terribly hurt. He began to hate his mother for running away from him. It took him years and years to forgive her even after he found out she'd really O.D.'d—committed suicide with an overdose of sleeping pills. And now, whenever he gets drunk, he starts thinking about his mother, he says, and then he feels angry and he wants to hurt somebody, especially somebody close to him. That's his explanation, anyway. But I don't care; it's not my fault that-

"Dr. Sherwood, what am I getting myself into? I came in here worrying about no orgasm, but I hear myself talking about Robert, and I realize he's really a troubled guy. I love him, but I keep wondering if he's really for me. He's got all the qualities I like in a guy. He's so handsome all my girl friends just ogle when they see him, and he's very intelligent, and he's going to be a brilliant lawyer someday. And he can talk about anything with me, almost. He can even be very sweet, till he gets one of his mean spells, and then he's terrible to be near. Thinking about that sends shivers through me, and I feel like vomiting.

"But I can't make up to him for what happened when he was a kid. I can't make up for her. I can't become his mother, I can't—"

She turned around and looked at me quizzically. "If I hadn't been in analysis I never would have thought of this. I never would have thought of this right now," she repeated. "I've been thinking and thinking about him for weeks, about his crazy, unreasonable angry spells, his testing me constantly and comparing me to his other girl friends to see if I'm loyal, his meanness about my not having an orgasm, as if I'm not responding to him, and his terribly frightening madness at his mother for letting him down, for not loving him enough because he felt he wasn't good enough to be loved by her.

"It sounds like psychiatric bullshit, but it's really true. I see it now. His taking it all out on me, unconsciously, when he's been drinking, or when he's stoned and his guard is down. It makes sense. They're all connected. He's always told me how terribly empty and lonely he feels when he thinks someone let him down, even if a boyfriend forgot to phone him on some minor matter like going to a movie. And if it's a girl friend who lets him down, he not only feels betrayed, he goes into a rage. It makes sense," she said. Her voice trailed off as she stared at the ceiling, forgetting momentarily where she was. "It all makes so much sense to me, now."

"Good," I said. "At last you're willing to examine what you've been dealing with for a long time. I said to you more than once, 'Look at your relationship with Robert. See what it signifies. See what his attack on you and your willingness to maintain this liaison with him means.' You've been aware for a long time that there was something deeply wrong with Robert's emotional makeup, but only you, Belinda, can make the choice of continuing or terminating your affair."

"I know," she said. "I know." Tears came to her eyes. "It hurts so much to think of giving him up. It hurts so deeply. I wish now I'd never met Robert; yet in a way I'm glad I have because it means that I'm able to have a relationship with him or with someone, at least. All these years of looking at myself have helped me"—then she laughed—"have helped me to be able to develop a new kind of misery. Lucky me. But I am different, so different from what I used to be. I can feel it. Yet I wish I'd never met him." Tears flowed down her cheeks as her laughter faded.

I looked at her, but I said nothing. Yet my mind was filled with thoughts:

I'm moved, Belinda, deeply moved by your pain. I am aware that I feel angry at Robert. How good is the bastard for you? He's inflicted a powerful emotional trauma on you, and he might upset some of the gains that you've made in your emotional development over the past four years. No, he couldn't undo your insights, or the long period of growth, but the SOB has stopped some of your momentum.

And now I realize that you have become more than just a patient. You have become, in part, my daughter, my lover, and maybe even my little sister, and these sometimes parts have grown too large for me. I've developed an affection for you as a person, a patient possession that I feel like protecting. My countertransference feelings, there they are again. There's no escaping them, is there? Yet is it really possible to be totally detached? No, not at all. A little proprietary interest is even good. It acts to stimulate my responses, but it's safe only as long as I stay aware of myself and keep analyzing my own feelings and never lose sight of them so that my analysis of you, Belinda, our mutual analysis of you will go on as objectively as psychiatrists-psychoanalysts can be objective.

Belinda, your unconscious seduction of me is the same behavior that you have directed toward all men, beginning with your father. Your cleverness, your humor, your attractiveness as a woman, and your bewildered girlishness are all present simultaneously in you. Your father wished to maintain, at least in part, your helpless state so that he might retain his role of indispensability. I was aware from the start that you could have that same effect on me. Still, at the very same instant that you unconsciously wish me to live out the role of your father, you remonstrate against me in that role, for it usurps your independence.

I'm also aware that some part of me has responded to your seductiveness and wishes to keep you dependent on me, making me delightfully needed and wanted and indispensable, as your father himself wanted to be, and omnipotent and omniscient to boot. But I have not and shall not yield to that desire, and the wish will shrink away.

Whether to keep or to reject Robert is your choice as you and he will have it. My only demand on you, Belinda, is to continue to dig into yourself, to be aware of your past and your present and never to cease learning about yourself and your reactions so that more of your future will be in your own hands.

A few weeks later Belinda entered with a twisted smile on her face I had never seen before, a mixture of anguish and triumph.

"Well," she said, "I finally had it—my first orgasm. I know what it feels like. I've never had anything like it before, and it was all the startling things, all the crazy pleasure, all the unbelievable feelings I ever heard about it. And it was with Robert. I should be happy about it, because I finally had one, and because I finally proved to him that I could have it, and to myself. But I'm not happy because—because Robert's gone. He left last night. We had another one of those bitter fights and he left on the night of my first orgasm. How's that for a date to remember?" She smiled that twisted smile again as if she were in pain. Then she opened her mouth as her tongue curled and straightened again and again inside it, in a gesture of which she was unaware.

She spoke sharply now. "I hate him, and I hate myself, and I hate you, and I hate everyone else!" She was about to scream, to volley forth a stream of tears, when she suddenly checked herself. Her face blanched. Her voice grew strangely quiet and controlled.

"It doesn't make sense. There's no point to this, crying and knocking myself out—no sense. He isn't for me! He just isn't! We'll never make it together and it's better for me—for us—to know it now. I asked him to move out of my apartment, and he's gone now. We're not living together any longer.

"Anyway, for weeks I've been thinking about it all, again and again—about Robert and me, and our whole relationship," she said slowly. "The tragedy of my little old orgasm is the least of my concerns now. It's Robert and me I'm thinking about—the whole relationship," she repeated. "I think it's too much like the way I was with my father nearly four years ago when I started my analysis. I had a need to cling to my father because he and I—we wanted it that way—not that he deliberately set out to make it that way, but that's how it turned out. He needed me for a substitute wife to use as a weapon—a power tool against my mother—and all the other reasons we've talked about. My father and I had what I see now was a strange, queer closeness, a tie that I couldn't break, or didn't want to—four years ago.

"That was a long time ago," she turned to look at me fully, "a lifetime, I think. Every time something went wrong I got sore at my dad the way I did at you just now, as if I expected him to make everything all right. And if he didn't, I held him responsible, and I hated him. I know that's crazy. I've known it now for a long time. And still for a minute just now I couldn't help it. I felt so rotten—the old feeling just came back to me again, this time toward you, the way it has sometimes before. And I know that's crazy too—my crazy transference—you don't have to tell me. I really know it."

There was a long, thoughtful pause. Now she spoke even more deliberately.

"I know I have to give Robert up permanently. I've been thinking about it for a long, long time. We've known each other over a year now—I mean really known each other, living together. I love him. But he's not for me. I can see it—he's got too many hangups. He says so, too. He's been thinking about analysis, he says, but he's too scared, and it's too much work, and it takes too long, and it costs too much. I told him to apply to the clinic of your Institute, but he's really afraid to, afraid of what he might find out." The shrill pitch of her voice, which long had been characteristic of her, was absent.

"But as long as he's that way, I can't go on being with him. He knows it, too. He gets these rages at me, then he's sorry, but he can't control them. So I just said we should break up. I have my teaching, and my girl friends, and my other social activities. I know I'll be terribly lonely at first, and I'll want to phone him, but I won't. I just can't. He's not good for me."

She began to cry softly. "He's just not good for me. I feel like dying. But there's no way I can live with him, no way." Then she startled me with a loud cry and began weeping heavily. Her face and shoulders shook spasmodically. After a few moments her sobbing died down. She groaned and said in a slow, husky voice, "No one, no one can tell me what to do, no one—neither you, nor my mother, nor my dad, nor my friends. I don't even ask my parents any more what I should do. I'm the only one who can decide.

"Sometimes I feel like running home again to mom and dad like a little girl. But I don't and I won't. So much else of my life is going so well. My teaching is fine. The kids love me. The second grade is so easy. I never dreamed I could make it, much less that I'd ever get to like it. For someone as mixed up as I was to get through school and get a teaching credential is a miracle. I was only going through the motions of going to college the first few years. I guess I always hoped that somebody would step in and take care of me—daddy or somebody; you know the story—and that I'd never have to do it myself. And here I am, at least pretty much unmixed now—stable—and still miserable."

She smiled sardonically as she spoke. "That's what psychoanalysis does for you. It helps you become stable while you're miserable so you can suffer in a more mature way."

She waited before going on. "And I did it all myself—with a little help from psychiatry. Great stuff, psychiatry. It helps you become grown up. But as you keep reminding me, Dr. Sherwood, I really did it all myself.

"But there really is something different about me, now. Even though I'm terribly depressed, I know I'll get over it. I won't fall to pieces. Robert isn't the only one I can fall in love with . . . I know. He's not the only one. I'm handling it. I've learned, and I know I can't and won't run home or call my daddy to take care of me.

"When my mother phones my apartment to ask what's going on, I know she and dad really are asking about Robert and me. But I tell her nothing. And when she keeps prying, I tell her if we're married she'll be the first to know. Then I hear her choking on the other end of the line and that shuts her up for the time being. And when my dad begins to work on me, I remind him of who I used to be, and who I am now, and who he is, and that if he wants to know about anyone's love life, to turn around and work on his own wife, not on me.

"Those days are gone, long gone. This is the new me, the thin me. I can take care of myself now, and I have my girl friends if I need someone else besides myself and my analysis. And as you said, I won't need this much longer either, because I know I can handle my life now, no matter what happens. I don't need another person to cling to, the way I did to my daddy all those years. If Robert isn't there to be in love with me, it will be someone else. I know it now," she said thoughtfully. "I have to try hard to forget him.

"There is this new guy I've been talking with lately." She brightened a little. "Another new teacher at school—very cute. But he's pretty shy. I can tell. He gets tongue-tied the way I used to. Either that, or I'd talk too much because I was so nervous. But he likes me. I know from the way he looks at me. It makes me feel good. So I have to keep the conversation going. Imagine. Me being the one who's calm and collected."

She smiled a little, though her face was wet with tears. "Well, this new guy who's so shy he gets upset when he's near me—I think he was trying to ask me for a date when I had to tell him where the men's john was, he was so flustered, so he wouldn't poop in his pants. I think he has a nervous bowel habit, the way I had," she laughed. "But I think I can help him." She smiled again.

"If he sticks with me, and doesn't give up, he can be helped," she said, looking at me as her smile saddened. Tears came to her eyes once more.

"I'm trying so hard," she said, looking at me again. "But I know it's the end—for us—for Robert and me. We've broken up for good— and on the night I've been waiting for all these years. It's so funny," she wept while she laughed, "all on the night of my first orgasm, when I finally knew I can be myself."

Chapter 5
Harry's Heart

Harry sat clenching his hands together and said, "I'm scared. I dunno why or how it began but I'm scared. My heart pounds and I think I'm gonna die of a heart attack! Dr. Bramovitz told me a dozen times it's just my nerves, but I can't believe him."

He held the left side of his chest with his hand, a half-smiling, half-anguished look on his face. "I just feel I'm gonna die. My heart begins to pound, and then I feel a funny sensation as if my heart stops; then it begins to pound again and the sweat breaks out all over me, and I just know I'm gonna die of a heart attack any minute."

I see the terror in his face! It's a round and full face, and his large, dark eyes are fixed on me as if to suckle courage from me even in the opening moments of our first meeting.

He nearly choked once or twice as he spoke, swallowing hard and licking his thick, dry lips with his tongue.

"I know it sounds crazy, but I checked with another doctor or two. In fact," he smiled, "five or six. You can see I don't take no chances. They all took cardiograms—is that what you call it?—and examined me, and all of 'em said the same thing—except one guy! I watched that doctor's face as he listened to me with his stethoscope. He looked grim. I looked down at him from his examining table, but he didn't say a word—not for a long, long time. Then all of a sudden he made a strange face like he was gettin' sick just listening, and I almost died right then and there. 'What's wrong?' I said, but he just kept listening and then he looked at the cardiogram again and then I really died.

"'Looks a little peculiar,' he said. 'T wave's a little flat.'

"By then I was flatter than any T wave that guy ever saw." Harry laughed slightly, his heavy frame shuddering. "Boy, if you think I'm scared now, you shoulda seen me then. 'What's that T wave mean, doctor? Tell me, quick!' My mouth was so dry I could hardly talk. I couldn't wait to hear.

"'We'll check it again in a couple of weeks,' he said. But I got out of there, and he ain't ever gonna see me again. Not him! I seen six doctors, and he's the only one who didn't tell me there was nothin' wrong after just a few minutes. I don't trust him." He laughed again.

It's an appeasing chuckle to assure me that his anger toward the doctor was reasonable, so that I won't destroy Harry with a diagnosis that he's deathly ill, as if I held his fate in my hands.

"Besides, I'm no fool! I'm not going back to no doctor who tells me I might be sick. The only doctor I want to see is one who tells me I ain't sick!"

"So Dr. Bramovitz sent you to me?"

"Yeah. He must think I'm sick too, but only in the head. Tell me at least I ain't crazy. I gotta have something good to think of tonight, especially after you tell me how much this is gonna cost me! But no, seriously, Doctor Sherwood, I'm really scared. I can joke and laugh 'cause I was a little bit in show business and I did some entertainin', a long time ago, but I ain't kiddin' you, the last few months has been hell for me."

He shifted in his chair, clutched his collar, and wiped his brow repeatedly.

That damned Bramovitz! He always sends me tough ones like this. Oh well, I've got to make a living! I'd better make a note to phone Bill Bramovitz to make sure this patient is telling me everything correctly. If I reassure him, he'll be content for as long as the ten steps out my door. Then he'll be scared stiff again. I've seen too many of these not to know this by now. And if I fail to say anything reassuring, he'll be more scared than ever—if that's possible.

"I've seen this problem before," I said. "It's not too uncommon." I knew others had already told him this.

His gaze pierced into me again. "You mean I'm not the only one who's worried like this? Thank goodness. I was so worried, Doctor, and now I'm relieved."

His large dark eyes looked up. "Thank God! I keep thinking I'm gonna die, and I just pray to heaven and hope He's up there listenin' to me. But you really think there's nothin' to worry about? I worry all the time, Doc, but I feel better now, much better. You come so highly recommended that I'm glad you could take me."

I see his face. It's changed back to what it was a moment ago. I was right.

He looked at me again, smiling meekly. "Are you sure there's nothing wrong with my heart? I know you want to talk to my doctor first, but you're an M.D., too. Do you think there could be something wrong? Ask Doctor Bramovitz to tell me the truth—or maybe better not to—I don't want to hear it. Let him tell you. I'm so worried." Again he placed his hand over his heart. "Jeez, am I worried!"

It was really so much easier as a G.P. "Take these pills and go home and relax—one every four hours." At least this guy has a sense of humor. That should make the sweating easier for me. And why should I be that concerned anyway?—because I always need to succeed? My mother loved me enough, my analysis showed, so that I could endure failure too. Be brave, you ass, treat him! And have less therapeutic ambition. Boloney! We all have that ambition. Freud himself, genius that he was, was at times defensive against failure. But how much can I demand even of a Freud?

"I'll see you and we'll explore further, if you want to. Chances are that you might be able to feel much better if your trouble is essentially emotional. Let me talk to Dr. Bramovitz first and we'll meet another time. . . ."

A few days later we continued. "How does something like this even begin?" he asked. "I remember bein' scared before, but nothin' like this! I'm even scared of leaving home to go to work. I can't understand it, Doctor. My heart begins to pound the minute I get in my car, I'm so scared. When I think of drivin' all the way out to my dress store—Jesus, I get so scared!

"My wife says, 'Heck, you're OK. Go to work. Don't worry so much.' And I love her for it. She tries to encourage me, but when I see her close that front door after she says goodbye, I feel like a kid who's been locked out of his home and who's gonna break down and cry.

"Jesus! I say to myself, God! Pull yourself together—you're a man! You're forty-six years old—nothin' is gonna happen to you." Tears came to his eyes.

"Nothin' is gonna happen, I keep telling myself, but I don't believe nobody, especially me." He looked anxiously about the room.

"How long have you felt like this, Harry?" I asked. "This intensely, I mean."

"Just the last few weeks, Doc—maybe a couple of months. Oh, don't get me wrong. I was never a General George Patton. I always been a little scared, but nothing like this. Now I'm goin' outa my mind. This thing is driving me crazy! I hope you don't have to send me to the loony bin! Jeez. Someone, I think it was my sister-in-law, mentioned the hospital! That's all I had to hear!" He slapped his cheek. "Then I really panicked. Jesus! The hospital! A customer o' mine said her husband's been in now for over four years. Four years! The way she talked, he's a goner—been in a state hospital most of that time 'cause they started to run out of money, and his psychiatrist advised her not to sell her house just to raise cash for private care, 'cause he said it wouldn't pay off. So they transferred him to a state hospital. Jesus. Does that scare me!"

He paused, waiting for a reply.

What a hysteric! The loony bin! Damn, I should be more understanding! He's really scared of the loony bin. Did I ever in my life have such severe anxiety? Is it what I felt going uphill against the krauts with the eighty-eights whistling in? I remember how hard my heart beat when I had the gasoline tanks on my back the night we were going to jump off to surprise them and I "knew" I'd be incinerated.

And when I was a kid, sometimes I had terrible fears when I realized that someday I would die. And then there was my fear of never being accepted to a medical school when I'd worked so hard for it so many years and it meant so much, as if my life were at stake, the long moments of panic despite everyone's reassurance that I would surely make it. That's how he must feel about losing his mind or dying when his heart begins pounding and he doesn't know why.

"Her husband's problem," I said, " may have been entirely different from yours, Harry. We've got to know more about what's behind yours."

"You mean if we find out the thing that's botherin' me, I'll feel good again?"

"No, it's not that simple. That's only in the movies. But it's important for us to find out all we can about your scared feelings and what set them off." Then I explained that "free association" would be our method of approach.

Best for him not to lie on the couch. He's much too anxious and troubled for that. He needs direct contact with me. He understands my explanation and seems bursting to continue.

"I'll tell you the truth, Doc, I always been a worrier. I can remember worryin' about my health even years ago before I was married. I used to travel a lot when I was a kid in my early twenties. I did nightclub work. This was a long time before I got into the clothing business, ladies' clothes, that I've been in for these last sixteen or seventeen years, and I remember always thinkin': What if I got sick in Chicago or Kansas City, real far from home? Who could I phone? Who could I go to? I always worried about gettin' sick. Then I'd forget about it for a few days when I got used to a new place. When we moved on to a new town, I'd get scared all over again."

He clenched his hand into a tight fist and thumped his chest. "I always put on a good front and joked a lot and laughed, but I'd always make sure someone in the company looked after me—like the lady singer, or a member of the band, or my manager, or someone in the hotel—like jokin', I'd say to them, 'Come on over after the show or give me a ring, huh? Just in case, 'cause I'm all alone tonight.'

"'Just in case what?' they'd ask me, laughin'.

"'Oh, you know, just in case,' I'd say, and someone would always come look in on me.

"Gee, I remember, around the time when I was still new in show business, something that must be important. It comes back to me now. I was only about twenty-one or twenty-two. We were in the Catskills playing one of them little places in the borsht belt. My act was on. Things were going good when all of a sudden a guy keels over in the audience near the back. I hear a commotion and they're carrying this man out, see? I could spot him from the stage, and the audience got all upset and everyone was talkin', interruptin' my act. I kept right on with my jokes, but from then on I couldn't keep my mind on my work. He wasn't an old guy—maybe in his fifties, slightly grey. I could see them carrying him out, and it ruined my act, and damm it, that night the audience was eating me up, and then that hadda go happen. I began to shake inside. And I began to lose my delivery—you know, the punch was gone—but I kept up with my act.

"Just as I was finishing, I heard someone up front say, 'He's dead— the man they carried out is dead!' Then I had to leave right away! I didn't wanta stay in that nightclub any more, no matter what, even though they loved me. And we had three more days scheduled there. I just wanted to get out of there. My manager pressured me real hard to stay, but I didn't feel like it. I was scared every night I went on for the next few nights—like I was always expectin' someone in the audience to keel over, and my jokes came on bad after that."

"Did you find out what really happened to the man?"

"Oh, he honestly did die, I heard. I don't know what from—heart attack I guess. But I kept seeing them carrying him out of there, and I kept thinkin' it could someday happen to me.

"And later on word got around that he was all alone when he came to the hotel that night."

The patient began to weep suddenly, bending over in his chair and burying his black, curly head in his arms. "I kept thinkin' of that poor guy, all alone, being carried out of the nightclub— nobody knowin' who he was—not even the broad who was with him.

"I imagined that maybe he picked her up that night at the bar 'cause he was lonely, and maybe he wanted to get laid, too—but I—"

His weeping began anew, and he looked up at me, as if expecting disapproval for his tears. I nodded for him to continue.

"The poor guy reminded me of my father, all alone." His voice broke. "All alone after my mother divorced him. We were just kids when she decided to leave him. I remember hearing him plead with her before she kicked him out. He even—Jeez, I remember—he even cried like a lost kid the night she finally decided to break it off.

"When we were young, they never got along, always quarrelin' and bickerin' year in, year out. Finally, she decided she had to divorce him. I was twelve, my kid sister just turned ten, my little brother about eight. What a lonely feeling I had for him. I couldn't believe she really would do that to him. You know, families quarrel and fight, but they didn't separate, at least not in them days.

"I felt so sorry for my dad, even though I really never felt close to him. He was such a pitiful character—never had any skills, except maybe sellin' things. For a long time he sold brushes and combs and floor polish and little things from door to door. Sometimes I'd go with him after school, and I'd watch the look on his face when the people who answered the door would say, 'No, we don't need nothin' today,' or they'd slam it in his face. And he would walk away with his head down, light up a cigarette, and start coughin'. He was always coughin' from smoking so much.

"'It's OK, Pop,' I'd say. 'Heck, let's go on. Someone else will buy from you.' But sometimes nobody'd buy all day, and he'd go home with all his suitcases full of brushes and things, just like he hadn't been out selling.

"And when he'd get home, my mom would give him hell. 'Look at mine peddler! *Schlemielidiche*, old *Yid!*' she'd say.

"Yeah, that's right. She was Jewish herself and she'd call him that! He was a lot older than she was.

"How come, I used to wonder, she married a guy like that? She was tall and slender, and people used to tell her how pretty she looked. How come, I used to say to myself, she married a *schlemiel* like my father—didn't have much schoolin', didn't have no profession—and she would *hok* him, day after day, that he wasn't much good, couldn't make a livin' for his family, and how she shoulda' married someone who would've amounted to somethin'.

"That would make him real mad, and he'd say he was trying his hardest, and he'd swear at her and call her a husband-killer—and then she would tell him how sorry she was she married him and how she shoulda left him years ago. Then he would be afraid to say anythin' more 'cause he was scared she would really leave, and the poor guy had to keep quiet so as not to antagonize her more.

"I felt so bad for him. Bein' the oldest, I was the only one of us kids who really knew how he felt. And I was only twelve years old. Each time he couldn't make a livin' at a new job, it would get worse, and they would quarrel, and she'd call him 'dumb' and 'no good.' It was still during the depression, you know. Finally, she herself got a job as a beauty operator. I don't know what right she had to criticize my father, 'cause she had such little education herself. But she did fairly well. And he felt terrible, seein' his wife going to work every day to make ends meet and seein' his kids come home after school with no mother around, and we hadda make the meals and clean up the house.

"And my dad looked worse and worse, 'cause then his cough got real bad. In fact, once, just before they split up, he went into the hospital. 'Emphysema' is what the doctors said he had, from smoking. I could tell how frightened he was, 'cause he couldn't catch his breath and he felt so alone. My mother really wasn't interested in him anymore. And the other kids, they were too young, and later they didn't care about him either. But I knew how he felt. He told me that he didn't want to split up with my mother, never, but she wanted to.

"But there were times when I really wanted them to live apart 'cause they were always bickerin' and fightin' and it made life so unpleasant, but then again, I really didn't want them to 'cause I knew how lonely he'd feel.

"Finally they decided to split up. I'll never forget it.

"For days he moped around and looked so sad before he left. He was really gettin' sick by then. The day he left, he couldn't even carry his suitcases up the rickety stairs of that dinky little third-floor apartment he moved to just a few blocks from where we were living in Brooklyn 'cause he was so short of breath and tired. I went with him to help him move. I said, 'Here, Pop. Let me do it.' And I carried his baggage up. And once I got them upstairs, he just sat there on top of his suitcases, cryin'. And that's where he lived till the time he passed away."

He's working well, Harry, better than I expected. And he has depth. He can grow even with his apparent simplicity. Once I believed that only a few of us on earth could understand enough to really matter. Are most people as egocentric as I was? Or was it just my need to see myself as exceptional? He's struggling so damned hard to be in control despite his fears. I'll push him hard to explore his childhood. That's where many of the secrets lie, I suspect, the "secrets" that blossomed into his terrible anxiety.

"I was telling you about my pop last time, and I remember my mother never encouraged us to go visit him, so I'd sneak off after school. And I'd find him home alone—all by hisself, sittin' there readin' a newspaper or just sittin', 'cause he worked in the mornings.

"'Hiya, Pop,' I'd say, 'cause I wanted to cheer him up a little bit. He said I was a good boy." His voice broke, "'Cause I worried about him and no one else did. But I never really loved him—just felt sorry for him—always with that sad look on his face. He never smiled.

"But after a year or so my dad surprised us all and got married again to a widow who moved into his building just two months before. He was that lonely. My mother said the *yenta* he married musta' thought he had some money hidden away—else why would she marry a sick old man? By then he was grey and thin and all hunched over.

"I remember visiting them a few times. I can vaguely remember— his new wife seemed awfully strange. She was thin and had a long nose, hardly said anythin', never had been married before, almost never left their apartment. Even my dad felt she was odd 'cause he whispered to me one time that she was a *miesse*, the 'ugly strange one,' but she did his cookin' and cleanin' and helped him live a little easier. He knew he didn't have much longer to go. And after another year or so he grew worse and ended up in the county hospital. He actually had no money. And there wasn't much they could do for him anyway. And then I learned his new wife left him too—she didn't count on him bein' that sick.

"Jeez! Just thinkin' about it, I start to grow short of breath." He looked up in embarrassment and tried to smile, but his look of fear sprang back.

I feel his pain and his struggle to control himself again.

"Then one day when I came home from school, my mother was all dressed up. 'Your father's pretty sick,' she said. 'A nurse phoned and said he asked for you.' My heart pounded, I remember. And the reason, Doc, that I remember so good is that I heard that the doctors thought he had a strong heart. Otherwise, he'd a' been dead long ago. So there was a lot of emphasis on heart.

"Am I doing OK, Doctor? You said I should look into myself and how come I have all these worries about myself and gettin' sick and all and I'm lookin'—and I think I'm findin' out 'cause it's comin' back to me now."

"Yes, you're doing well. Go on."

"So we went to the hospital, just me and my mother. The other kids were too young. And I went into his room. His new wife was called, too, 'cause there she was. She saw my mother and said hello, and they were both there, his old wife and his new one. And neither one wanted him—they just came 'cause—'cause—" He covered his face as the tears rolled down. "Excuse me, Doc."

"It's OK."

He swallowed hard. " 'Cause he was dyin'. And my mother told me his new wife wanted to get whatever money she could. So she came to the hospital to prove she had a right to his belongings.

"And there he was—in an oxygen tent, gaspin' and tryin' to breathe. His lips were blue, and I could tell, even as a kid, he was a goner. The whole bed shook every time he sucked in another breath. He saw me and tried to say somethin', but he couldn't get the words out. . . ."

Harry broke off and wept openly, bending over and putting his head in his arms. He tried to continue, but his sobbing choked off his words.

"There he was. I'll never forget it. Him fightin' to breathe, and I said to myself, so that's how it is when you die. And I just had to get outa there—I couldn't take it. I just had to get out of the room. So I left him there, dyin', with his new wife and his ex-wife at his bedside, but really all alone 'cause neither one cared for him or wanted him.

"Later on my mother said he reached out to take her hand, but he couldn't say nothin'. She said he didn't even look at his new wife, but I can't be sure 'cause my mother exaggerates—you know how it is. She was the only one he ever loved, she told us."

"What happened? Your father didn't make it through that day?"

"No—no, he didn't. I went outside with my mother to get some fresh air, and an hour later we came back. I was still panicky. I wanted to see him 'cause he really was all alone, but I just couldn't go back into that room. I waited outside debatin' with myself. And finally the nurse came out and said he was gone."

He bowed his head, his face serious.

"Sometimes when I get my anxiety attacks, for a second I see my father lyin' there coughing and fightin' to breathe—my heart starts pounding and missing beats; I break into a sweat; and I feel like I might die any minute, too. I never realized it before, strange as it seems, but when that picture starts to come to me I push it right out of my mind. I guess I really feel like I'm him. But I push the whole thing out of my mind." He waved his arm out in front of his body. "And then the picture's gone, but I'm still short of breath and feel like I'm goin' to die, but I forget that he came to mind—like I don't want to remember it."

"You push the picture of your dying father out of your mind, but the feeling you have stays on?"

"Yeah, that's right. Sounds crazy. I just push it outa my mind. Maybe 'cause I don't want to think I could ever be like him. Yet, I'm afraid I really am. My mother always felt he was such a 'weak man,' she would say. Weak 'cause he was always afraid to try things out in business or to talk to people—like when the landlord came to tell about raisin' the rent, he'd hide out and make my mom face the landlord to try to argue him out of it. He was shy and scared and I tried to be more like—like—" His voice broke again, "Like, I guess, the kind of man my mother wanted, aggressive and not afraid of people, someone who could talk. Maybe that's why—hey! Maybe that's why I went into show biz, 'cause as a kid I always tried to be funny and talk to a lot of people, like my mother wanted, and she would smile and say, 'Harry's gonna be a good businessman someday. He knows how to talk to people.' And she was so proud of me.

"And I hated to think I could be anythin' like my father—scared and weasel like. I used to pity him. I didn't want to be like him, yet I was so scared that I would be.

"Yeah, I'll bet that's one reason I did try out as an entertainer. I was good, too, except when the audiences started gettin' bigger. Then I'd start to think of myself as bein' small like my dad and less able to talk—and I'd feel tight and I—I guess maybe I'd think, how could I make all them people out there laugh?—little me—and I'd get scared to talk to them. Gee! I never thought of that before! That's really so, I think. With small audiences I'd feel at home—I'd have them layin' in the aisles. Big audiences were like the big people to my dad and me— I'd get real tight inside."

"So," I said, "one of the unconscious motives behind your becoming an entertainer was your wish to be able to overcome your fears of people by charming them, thereby getting the confidence to be able to speak openly and aggressively to them, in order to gain control over them, and finally to stick the shaft to them through humor, to prove to yourself that you had a pair of balls—unlike your dad."

"Yeah. That's right. I did use sarcasm a lot, and I did kid the audience about themselves all the time, like I was on top, and they were just there to be kidded. I'd pick people out in the audience and ridicule them, and when I got them laughin' at each other, I'd feel good, and then I had 'em eatin' outa my hand. I started makin' good, and I got bookings at the big hotels like the Mayfair and the Hilton. Then I'd get scared and my manager would say, 'How come you came over so stiff tonight?' The big hotels never asked me to come back.

"But gettin' back to those anxieties, Doctor. Bein' scared of sickness didn't just come from my father's dyin'. I remember being scared long before that."

"That's right. I guess that your father's death just fed the fears you already had inside of you and helped them grow. No single incident accounts for all symptoms—except maybe in the movies."

"Yeah. Like my idea if I could only find out the one thing that's worryin' me, I'd be all right. I can see already it just don't work like that.

"But I'm glad I could go over my dad's dyin', 'cause I could never really look at the whole thing before—not in the open like this and face it."

"You tend to become overwhelmed by anxiety, Harry. You become buried by your worries even if they're small, as if there is no way in the world of finding a solution to any problem—the same as you must have felt as a kid. But you're working well now, and what really counts is an understanding of what makes you tick, the unconscious and conscious factors, and what you can do to be different."

"Can a guy really change, Doc—I mean can a person really become different?"

"No question," I said. "If he really wants to work on it."

"I sure do," he said.

Occasionally I summarized for Harry the content of our meetings of the past few weeks or month.

"Like you say," he'd answer, "I gotta keep lookin' at things from different angles, even if we go over the same things ten dozen times. It begins to mean something when I keep lookin' and thinkin' about it, like learning how to feel about somethin' all over again. And maybe just knowin' you understand me helps, like you believin' in me, believin' that I can change."

"That's right, Harry, damned right."

When I felt I too could change, I changed. And when I felt my psychoanalyst was the kind of guy I wanted to be, I become more like him. I sensed how he felt inside of himself and then soaked up some of him and his values, the ones I wanted, inside of me. It happened unconsciously, at first. Later on, I became aware of it. It's happening to Harry, too. It'll lessen that tough conscience he has. I hope he keeps working on himself, just keeps working and never stops.

"I'm tryin' hard," he continued. "But sometimes it's so tough to be different. I get up in the mornin' and I feel scared, but I force myself to go to work, like you said. I don't stay home sometimes like I did before I saw you. But it's very tough on the mornin's when I'm real scared."

He rubbed his knuckles.

"I been thinkin' of what you said about explorin' myself and how I got this way, bein' I'm such a tense, worrisome guy, and some things begin to make sense to me. My mother played a big role in my fears.

She never let me think I could come out of any sickness without her there to help me—ya know, 'My chicken soup will help you better'n any doctor ever could,' she practically said. She thought she knew what to do better'n any doctor, if I ever had a fever or got sick. And I gotta confess, when all these fears began, I ran to her first, and I'd been callin' her every day, three and four times, for her to tell me what to do and to tell me everything'll be OK, same as when I was a kid, and she kept sayin' I don't need no psychiatrist—all I need is faith in her, and in myself, and I'll get over it.

"'Come on over,' she says, 'I got something good for you to eat.'" He laughed. "'You'll feel better.' She can always do things like no one else can, even better than the Lord, almost. She's like the tailor in a little tailor shop. Someone heard he was good and asked him to make a new sport coat. 'It won't be ready for thirty days,' the tailor said. 'Thirty days!' the customer yelled. 'Why, the Lord created the entire world in only six.' 'True,' said the tailor, 'but have you taken a good look at it lately?'

"But seriously, Doc, my mother always tried to make me feel I couldn't get along without her. Even before she divorced my dad, she was that way. Always givin' me advice and tellin' me what to do—it got so I relied on her alone to make my decisions, and she always pointed out how I would do well when I grew up 'cause I'd learn from her and not be like my dad who never did anythin' right.

"But my kid brother just didn't pay no attention to her. He laughed at her all of his life, and they used to quarrel 'cause he made fun of her and said she was crazy 'cause she said, 'If you're good to your mother, God will be good to you, and you'll be successful.' He even said, 'God's crazy, too,' and that really made her mad. So what does he do today, my brother?" He chuckled. "He's president of the Bank of America, and I was the one who was so good to her.

"I remember how she told me I was the oldest son, and 'cause I was so handsome and smart, it was God's way of givin' her somethin' good in life. She depended on me so much. Even as a little kid I began to worry about bein' successful. My brother and sister played the way ordinary kids do, but I'd sit at home doin' the chores, runnin' to the grocery, or helpin' her wash the floors and vacuum the house, and I kept thinkin' God would be good to me and make me successful.

"My mother seemed to leave the other two kids alone, but she always asked me to do things with her—go places and meet her friends, she was so ashamed of my dad. So when she would go to play bridge in the evenin' with her friends, she took me along to show off to them. And I'd dress up in my good suit. Funny. I never thought of it much before, but I was just like a little husband to her." He laughed. "Yeah, like a replacement for my dad. And all the women would make over me.

"She never tried it with my brother, 'cause he mocked her and poked fun at her and did everythin' bad, just to tease her. And, come to think of it, he really was jealous of me 'cause I was her favorite—more than just the oldest son—I was the old man! Maybe that's another reason why he began to hate her so much, 'cause as he grew up he always wanted to leave home, and they'd fight, and he'd swear at her and say she was 'an old Jewish bitch who tried to live everyone's life for him.' He actually married a gentile girl, sayin' he didn't want a loud-mouth Jewish dame like his mother for a wife.

"Reminds me," he smiled, "of when my mother warned my brother that if he married a gentile girl and she gets sore at him, she'll call him a 'dirty Jew.' I said to my mother if he married a Jewish girl, like my wife, and she gets sore at him, she'll call him everythin' *but* a dirty Jew."

He paused, thinking.

"Yeah, I was my mother's favorite. My kid sister didn't pay no attention to my mother, either. Funny how different kids can be.

"I was the 'chosen one.'" He smiled. "Like my own son. He's the chosen one, too—by me."

"What do you mean?"

"I guess I expect as much from him, even though he's only thirteen, as my mother wanted from me. I begin to find fault with him, like he isn't smart enough in school, and he can't play ball good enough, and like he's a sissy. I want him to be good in everythin', and I get after him. I don't want him to be shy or quiet like a *nebish*—I want him to be outgoing, just like my mother wanted from me." He smiled knowingly. "Just like my mother wanted me to be."

"So your wishes for your son became the same as your mother's wishes for you."

"Yeah, that's right. I guess my son has to live up to a lot of the things she wanted from me. Funny, I never looked at it that way before—that it's really what she wanted of me that I later wanted of myself that makes me so tough on the kid. I'm both the mother and the kid. Hey. That's really somethin'. I never really looked at it like that before!

"My wife always says to me, 'Don't be so tough on him. So he ain't gonna be a good ball player or tell jokes like you. He's a different sort of kid.' I want him to be a real excellent student in school—I wasn't bad—but I want him to be real good so he could become a professional, maybe a lawyer, or an engineer, or even a doctor. If he becomes a psychiatrist, boy, look at the money I could save!" He looked up with a grin that faded quickly. "I guess I really want to continue in him what my mother expected of me.

"When he plays ball and he drops it, I call him a 'butter-fingered sissy' and laugh at him."

"As if you wanted him both to succeed and to fail," I said.

"Huh? Maybe."

"Otherwise, why would you laugh at him?"

"Maybe you've got somethin' there, 'cause I know with my little brother, I'd laugh at him, and I knew I wanted him to be lousy so I could look better. So you mean my son is like both my son and my kid brother?"

"In your feelings, they may be one and the same. That's what I mean by the unconscious. Past attitudes come up again and again. You act like a stupe, sometimes, but that's deceptive. You're really a very clever guy. In business you're a shrewd cookie. You can outsmart all your competitors. But you have an emotional block, a blindness that prevents you from seeing in yourself what seems so obvious. You push back, away from awareness, the painful self-observations that would let you see yourself. In part, you are your mother, your father, and your son's brother.

"To be your mother's favorite," I continued, "you had to demean your kid brother, and now unconsciously you're doing the same with your son and your wife—as if you're again struggling to be the favorite son to your wife without being aware of the struggle. Another way of handling these troublesome feelings is to be funny, entertaining, clever—you became so good at it you even developed into a professional comedian. It's a good disguise to keep your hostility and jealousy from yourself and from the world. All that comes through to yourself is your anxiety. This has been hard for you to see, Harry, even harder to swallow, but you're beginning to."

Harry looked up at me with a smile of satisfaction. "I'm even beginnin' to feel a little bit less scared, too," he said.

I'm sugar-coating the bitter insights. That way he'll find them more palatable. He's doing well.

Harry continued, "I know I didn't want my brother to do well.

Every time him and my mother battled, I was a little glad, 'cause I knew she would bring up my name and praise me 'cause I was so good. Then I began to get sick of their quarrelin'. I hated to hear it year in, year out.

"I just realized something, right now. The better I became, the worse he grew. He began to hate me, too, and as he grew worse, I grew better. I did everything my mother wanted of me, and I'd get all the praise, and my poor brother couldn't do nothin' right. The better my grades were in school, the less he'd try, even if he flunked—he just gave up. My mother sees only two kinds of kids—good and bad—and I realize just now he couldn't win. So out of frustration he would be bad in school, tell the teachers to go fuck themselves, or he'd get into a fight with some kid and be sent home."

"I've seen this before," I said. "The split in feelings between two kids grows as each one unconsciously strives to live up to his label. Your brother behaved as if to say, 'If you think I'm not good, I have no chance. To hell with you! I give up, and I'll show you how really rotten I can be. And that'll hurt you just as much as you hurt me.'

"You, living up to your label of being the 'good' one and trying to avoid as much as possible getting kicked around like your father and catching hell like your brother, and to get every morsel of the love available, fought hard to be the better one. Underneath, you realized that your mother's contempt for your father, which had also turned upon your brother, could eventually fall on you. You struggled to stay at the opposite pole."

"Yeah, yeah, sounds right," he began thoughtfully. "I guess my own kid is competition to me, like you say. Yet I see myself in him and I want him to succeed, but maybe somehow I don't want him to make me look too bad—I want everyone to see me as a successful businessman, though business ain't so good lately. If my Ronny becomes a lawyer, look how much ahead of me my kid will seem—a college graduate—everyone will look up to him, and even I'd have to consult with him and ask him questions about leases and about business deals that I can't answer myself, like I do my own attorney now. And I would like it, except some part of me would be jealous, 'cause he made it and I didn't. Hmm. I think you've got somethin' there. Really. That's why I been so rough on him, even though consciously I'm all for him."

He looked down and stared at the floor for a while without a word.

"You know, I'm glad we're talkin' about this here, even if this ain't why I came in originally. Talkin' about everything that comes to mind about my life is good for me and my family too, 'cause I always knew I was too rough on the kid and I wanted to stop, but I couldn't. Now this finally came out o' me too. It always worried me."

That's what sugar-coating can do. Good. He sees that part of himself. I'll let him go on.

"My wife would say, 'You make Ronny feel bad about hisself, like he can't think for hisself. Don't blow up when he can't figure out a math problem right away. Give him a chance. You're givin' him a big inferiority feelin'. No wonder he has such a tough time makin' friends in school. He don't think much of hisself.' And, by God, she's right. I've been very tough"—his voice faltered—"very tough on Ronny, even slapping him around when I was mad at him, sometimes—as a little kid." Tears filled his large black eyes. He swallowed and looked up, wordless for a few moments.

"Yeah, I'm beginnin' to put the pieces together, like you say."

Harry began speaking before he sat down.

"You know, I been thinkin' more and more of my mother and why I get these heart poundings and how come I'm so scared and so dependent on someone like you for reassurance. Now more and more things come back to me. My mother really did want me to be dependent on her. She didn't even want me to get married or even go with girls who might marry me. When I came back from vaudeville and started opening my first clothing store, she was so happy. 'My Harry's come back to live with me in New York,' she said.

"She never liked it when I was gone, though she was hopin' I'd make it big in show business, like Eddie Cantor or Jack Benny maybe. Then she'd really been proud of me. She wanted me to live in her apartment with her and my kid sister, who was just about twenty and not married yet. And like a fool I came back. My kid brother was long gone—she wasn't even sure where he was livin' in the Bronx, 'cause he wouldn't tell her. And I opened my first store and, lucky, it did real well.

"Then I began dating a lot of different girls, and sometimes I'd bring them to the house, and afterwards she'd say, 'That one! She's too dumb, and this one ain't pretty enough, and that one's too fast for you,' as if I didn't know who was fast and who wasn't. I'd been around a bit—you know how it is in show business. Finally I met my wife, and I went with her quite a few months, and we started thinkin' of gettin' married. I was already twenty-six or twenty-seven and still livin' at home. When my mother saw me gettin' serious over one girl, she started sayin' she was getting older and maybe wouldn't be around a lot longer, and she started me worryin' about her, like thinkin' she might be sick and not tellin' me.

" 'No,' she said. She'd been to the doctor and everything was OK, except maybe she had a 'little trouble.' And I started thinkin', maybe she's got cancer or heart trouble and ain't tellin' me. I remember how scared I got. My imagination started runnin' wild. I even worry about cancer myself now, too. But I remembered how my poor father died, and I started seein' my mother lyin' in bed the way he did, and just thinkin' about it now my heart starts poundin'.

"So I worried about it. And the longer I went with one girl, the more I heard about my mother's 'little trouble.' She'd go to the doctor and always let me know about it, like, 'Don't worry; he says I'm really in good health, except for that little trouble with this and that, nothing too serious.' And now I know she really wanted me to call him, and not tell me herself, 'cause I'd really worry more about it if the doctor told me somethin' was wrong with her. She knew I'd call him. So I finally phoned without my mother knowin' it, and the doctor told me she's got a little high blood pressure, nothin' more.

"And I realized that she wanted me to worry and to stay at home with her and not get married yet. Almost like she said, 'I didn't remarry when you were a kid in order to take care of you, and you gotta do the same for me.' I see it now. She didn't say it in words, but that's what she meant. She didn't worry about my kid sister when she got married and moved out of our apartment—didn't make a fuss, even liked her son-in-law, she said. So just me and my mother were living there alone now.

"But with me, she looked over every girl I brought home. Once I went with a blonde showgirl that I really liked when I was still goin' with my wife before we were married. My wife and I had a quarrel, see, and we broke up for a few weeks. She wasn't smart, like my wife is, but real pretty and a sweet girl. Then my mother asked me if the new blonde is Jewish and I said, 'No, she's a shicksa.'

"That's when my mother's high blood pressure began to get worse. She'd say, 'Don't worry—just a little headache I got. Don't stay home for me.' So I could see her sittin' alone in her apartment, just like my poor old pop when he was alone. And I'd go out and I'd worry about her being alone, or I'd visualize her droppin' with a heart attack or rupturin' a blood vessel in her brain and keeling over dead, like I read in a medical book.

"I bought a bunch of medical books recently," he laughed, "hopin' my son would pick 'em up and get interested in medicine.

"So I couldn't enjoy the date thinking about my mother, and I'd come home early every time. So I guess that's another reason I worry about her heart attacks. My mother made me worry about her. I could sometimes see her lyin' there, like my father all over again."

"Then it was far more than just your father's terrible loneliness and illness and death that haunted you," I said. "Your earliest fears of getting sick were developed during your childhood, worrying about your father. In later years your mother, who already had a strong grip on you emotionally, began to work on your fears of illness all over again in order to get an even better hook onto you. What a trap you were in."

"Yeah, even the reason I broke up with my wife-to-be those few weeks had to do with my mother. My wife said she was always interferin' and doing everything but coming along on our dates.

"'Maybe she wants to do that too,' my wife says. So I jokingly said, 'That's a good idea. I'll ask Mom to come along to the dance next Friday.' But my wife didn't think it was funny." He grinned. "And she broke off with me and said she's not datin' me again till I tell my mother what's what. I stubbornly said I wouldn't tell mother nothin'. And I tried to make her jealous, so I started dating the shicksa and I began likin' her too. Then my mother really panicked."

"Your mother may not have been aware of how tightly she clung to you."

"Yeah, I think you're right. 'Cause she did it even on my wedding night. Remind me to tell you next time. Oh boy. Wait'll you hear that one. You won't believe it.

"But before I go today, I gotta tell you. I been feelin' better these past couple weeks. I been in therapy now a few months and, except for lapses now and then, I been feelin' much better. I keep thinking of what we talk about—goin' over it again and again in my mind—how I learned to be scared from my mother and her attitudes—how she really wanted me to stay scared and dependent on her, except she wasn't aware of it herself 'cause it has unconscious with her, for the most part—right? 'Cause she really needed a husband or some kind of man, and she used me as if I were her husband. And she divided me and my brother in her mind—everything good I was, and everything she didn't like about my father he became—in her mind." He paused for a moment, "And she caused my kid brother to hate her, and the more he hated her, the more she wanted me to 'love' her, 'cause she was lonely, too. And my father, he played an important role, too. . . ."

Good. He's caught on. He's learned to search himself. It's taken hold of him. He's a miniature psychiatrist. He's starting to integrate, to relate past and present behavior, to search himself again and again and again. His very searching for insight makes him a different person from the blind man he was.

"What's that, Harry? I missed your last few words. I was thinking . . ."

"I just said, 'Pretty good for an amateur.'" He smiled. "But I'm really beginnin' to see things more clearly. And it's fallin' into place. Now I look at everythin' I do, and I just don't let myself feel the world is gonna end every time I hear about a sick person or every time some woman at one of my shops says my styles stink and she ain't going to buy from me. I won't starve! My business will go on."

"About my wedding night," Harry began. "I guess it's easier to tell you 'cause I feel more comfortable with you now. And every day I go to work, and my three stores are holding up, even if I've got lots of worries. And even if some of the scared feelin's come up, I still do what I have to, like you said.

"When I got married, I didn't have much money, so we decided to go on a little honeymoon—five days in New England by the sea. But the wedding would finish late Sunday evenin', and we figured we ought to spend the first night at home. We, I mean my mother, figured, 'cause she said that would make good sense and we'd be welcome.

"So on Sunday afternoon we went to the Temple to be married. We planned a small wedding, just a few close friends—like all my mother's girl friends and all her card party friends and all her whole side of the family. There was just barely room enough for a friend or two of my wife's and me, my mother let us know. I wasn't even sure there was enough room left for my bride. After the wedding my bride and I were suppose to sleep in my old room for just one night. Then it happened. Just as we were turning out the light, we heard my mother scream. We both ran out, me half naked in my pajamas, my whang hanging partway out, and there she was lying on the floor just outside our door. I thought maybe she was gonna die. And though I was real scared then, right now after all of our talks, it only makes me mad at her, thinkin' about it.

"She started talkin' in a daze like. My wife thought she was fakin', but I knew better, 'cause my mother was saying somethin' about me and the shicksa. 'What are you talking about?' I said to her. 'The shicksa and me broke up. I didn't marry the shicksa.' But she kept muttering in a daze like how she lost her son to the wrong kind of girl and how could this happen to her and how God musta punished her, and I kept trying to tell her I married my wife—the Jewish girl—and how the shicksa and me broke up long ago. I didn't tell her it was on account of her father said he didn't want any circumcised pricks around his house and especially inside his daughter.

"Finally she came to and got clearheaded and said she just fainted. My wife said she put the whole thing on. But why would my mother do that? We were already married! Especially, sayin' crazy things like not knowing who I married. I figured my mother was havin' a stroke. Then when the doctor examined her, after he finally came, he said she didn't have no stroke, just fainted.

"That's how our marriage began. My wife claims it's my mother's way of saying she didn't think my wife was any better than the shicksa. But even if my mother wasn't puttin' on an act and really got confused, she was saying what she felt down deep in her head—now I can call it the 'unconscious,' like you say. Either way, my mother was putting my wife down. Nothing is lower than being called a shicksa by my mother, 'cause it means not just a non-Jewish girl, but an ignorant kinda low-class whore. All gentile women are no good, according to my mother, especially a dancer in show business.

"Yet the shicksa was a sweet girl, much to my surprise. She wasn't a bad type, sleeping with all the guys, even if she was a showgirl. In fact, she was a nice kid, didn't sleep with anyone, not even me. I couldn't take her to bed no matter how hard I tried, and some of the girls we traveled with would get drunk and take on the whole band, even the instruments if we wanted them to. But this girl was quiet and sweet and pretty. Her mother died when she was just a kid of sixteen. She couldn't live at home 'cause her father was such a rough guy. Wouldn't let her date even though she was twenty-one. So she ran off to be a dancer, and that's how I met her. I looked her up at home after I quit the business. She had gone back to live with her dad. When she began to like me, she felt she had to introduce me to him. That's when he kicked me out."

He smiled. "She got guilty on account of she began to like a Jew, and had her father do the dirty work. She acted surprised and hurt when he kicked me out, but I think it was her unconscious that made her set me up for him, even though down deep she must have known how he would feel about her seein' me. She made her father 'solve her conflict for her'—like you say.

"I was puzzled why she didn't just tell him off then, but now I know she had the same problem with her dad that I got with my mother."

Session after session continued.

"I been comin' along real good these past eight or nine months since my therapy began. Once in a while I get scared again, and the pounding begins sometimes like at the beginning. I get so scared I think I haven't gotten anywhere. But then I start thinkin' all over again of what we talk about and I feel better, usually. I try to do what I'm suppose to do. No stayin' home, though I'd like to sometimes."

Another year passed, and Harry worked hard going over his life, past and present, in great detail. One day in midsummer I said, "You've been doing quite well over the last year or so, Harry. In a few more months it will be three years since we began."

"Yeah. I been feelin' much better lately, and even when I do feel anxious, I've learned how to fight it and not let it get a hold of me. Now I'm sure my feelings won't kill me. I know I'll never be that scared again. I think I've learned a lot, Doc, about myself—an awful lot."

"We could reduce to two sessions a week," I suggested, "and then see about stopping after a few more months if all continues to go well with you. You mentioned the possibility of stopping a few times already."

He rested his chin on his hand. His black eyes looked down, then finally up at me.

"I think I could cut down. I wouldn't want to stop just yet, though. But I been thinkin' about it for these last few months, like you say."

"You're always working at it, Harry, even when you're not here. And that's good. Keep it up, always, even long after we've stopped," I said.

And we continued with our sessions for the next few months.

One Monday morning just prior to our weekly Tuesday appointment, Harry phoned me. "Doctor? Is that you? My boy's going into the hospital unexpectedly, so I have to cancel tomorrow. They saw something on an X-ray of his leg. I don't understand what it is, but they're going to do a 'biopsy,' it's called. They're worried it might be cancer, even though the odds are it's just a bone cyst, whatever that is. They want to play it safe. Can a kid of sixteen get cancer? Tell me, Doc. That's unusual, isn't it?"

"I guess they want to be certain, Harry. When did all this come up?"

"I just now found out about it. My wife called me. I'm at my store. She took him to the doctor 'cause he's been complainin' of pain in his leg these last few weeks. He thought he hurt it playin' ball. So she took him to our doctor, who sent him to a bone specialist. He saw something in the X-rays and wants him in the hospital. So I'm going in with him to Mt. Sinai. I'm a little scared. You know how it is, though I ain't falling apart like I might have two years ago."

"I'll see you next week instead. Good luck," I said. "Please phone me if it's anything serious."

His dark eyes were fixed on me as he entered. "The biopsy showed cancer, Doctor. I wrote down the name." He held the paper in his hand, but he knew the name without looking at it. 'Osteogenic sarcoma,' it's called. I even learned to pronounce it right. Have you seen it before?"

"Yes, years ago at Childrens' Hospital."

"Well, I didn't need to phone you. Thought I'd tell you myself. They're gonna operate. I've had a dozen consultants look in on him. They've got to take off his right leg." He faltered. "Maybe all the way to the hip to prevent it from spreading."

There was a long silence. "I just can't believe this is really happenin' to me." Harry was grave. "A few weeks ago my kid was OK—now somebody says he's got cancer!" He paused again. "And you know, Doctor, scared as I am for my kid, I ain't in a panic over it. I been watchin' myself like you always told me to do. Rotten as I feel, I'm stickin' it out pretty good. Even though my kid is losing a leg."

Tears poured down his face. "But I feel so rotten for the kid. I'd do anything in the world for him not to have it, but I'm not even thinkin' I could get it, too, or thinkin' maybe there's something I did to cause him to have it. I know cancer isn't catching. I always used to worry about that, too, with heart attacks, like you know. I really feel so bad for the kid. And just when I'm beginning to have a better relationship with him. I understand him better because of all our talking here. Him and I are starting to do things together, and now this has to happen. But I don't have no heart pounding, 'cause I really ain't scared any more. Except for him—

"The last few days I been to the hospital day and night just lookin' at him—and talkin' to doctors. Me and my wife—we haven't slept."

What did this sweet, sorrowful hulk of a man do to deserve this? Fate is as brutally relentless as a Nazi S.S. after a prey. I've always detested mortal fate. It listens to no one. It has no tenderness or reason. I hate it even more now, even though I seemed to have avoided it, sidestepped it many times.

Harry, you've grown so much in the last few years. You're able to take this without being destroyed by it as you would have before. You suspect he's dying, just the same as I do.

"I'm terribly sorry about Ronny," I said.

"Yeah," he interrupted. "But I'm not going to fall apart. Maybe they can save his leg from just above the knee. They'll decide today and operate tomorrow—'cause the cancer is in the bone just above the knee."

His dark eyes were deepset in two hollows of grief, reddened and nearly unseeing. "My kid is really in bad shape," he wept. "They took his leg off all the way to the thigh."

"Yes, I know."

"Yeah, that's right. I forgot. My wife told me you called."

He looked down at the floor. "I can't believe it. My kid's got no leg, and they're not sure he'll really make it. That's the thing that's got me really worried. Only time will tell, they said. I kept asking the surgeons and pumpin' them for more information. But they say they can't be sure. They want to give him X-ray treatment and cancer medicines too. That means it's bad, don't it?" He didn't wait for a reply.

"I've cried all I can cry," he said, looking up. But more tears began to flow. "I still can't believe it," he said. A couple of weeks ago everything was goin' good in my life. After all this time things started goin' good for me—and then something like this has to happen. I just keep hopin' I'll wake up and all this will be nothin' but a bad dream.

"Huh! It's a funny thing. I just said 'like it's all a bad dream.' I had a dream last night, and I can understand lots of it even though it was all mixed-up-like. My kid, my poor kid, was either my kid or my little brother, and we were young again, only I was married at the same time, 'cause my wife was watchin' us. My kid and I were playin' ball, and he was doing real good and I was enjoyin' him. Then he started droppin' the ball all the time, and I kept encouraging him—never got mad at him like I used to. Then he threw the ball wild, and it broke a window in an old rickety apartment house and glass shattered everywhere. And my dad sticks his head out of the broken window and he waves to me and I see his face is still sad.

"'Hiya, Pop,' I yelled, and now I was a kid again, too, about eleven or twelve years old, and I started playin' ball. Then I took some of my dad's brushes and brooms from his old suitcase and started cleanin' up the glass, and lots of people looked at me and said how good the brooms and brushes were and wanted to buy 'em from him.

"Then my mother comes into the dream. She says, *'Gay aveck,'* and dumps all my pop's brooms and brushes out on the ground and sneers at him, and everyone laughs at him.

"Then everything changes and my mother is feedin' my kid some soup, like chicken soup. I smiled at her and said 'Go ahead; give it to him if it makes you feel better, but he really don't need none of it. Nature will heal him 'cause he's a healthy kid and he don't need none of your soup.' Now my kid seems about eleven, too, and I'm about the same age in the dream, like now I'm his father and a kid at the same time. And my kid stands up, a little wobbly at first, cause his legs, or maybe one leg, ain't so good. Then he starts runnin' off to school like he's a favorite of the teacher 'cause he's such a good student, and he runs into the schoolroom and his sixth-grade teacher smiles at him.

"When he turns around, he turns out to be my kid brother, still about the same age, and him and me play a game of bein' comedians and tellin' jokes into a microphone to an audience and laughin' like maybe we did when we were close and friendly for a short time, especially if my mother wasn't home to set us against each other. And we have lots of fun. And the grey-haired man who died in the Catskills, he was in the audience. Jeez, what a dream! Only he's alive and laughin' at our jokes and he stays without keelin' over. Then my brother says to me—I'm not sure what the words were—something like, 'There's no business like show business except slow business,' and he runs off, and from behind, I watch him run off real slow, limping on one leg. And in the distance he becomes my kid again, like when he was six or seven, runnin' around real good—his leg is OK, like when he was a little kid and just beginnin' to grow up.

"And he's havin' a good time, and he's just a little kid again, my Ronny, and him and I are also playin' show business and havin' fun—only this time we're back in my old home again when I was a kid, and then the dream is over.

"I kinda know what most of it means. Like I want him to be small again, my kid, so's I can start all over with him and have a better relationship. I'm enjoyin' him and bein' the kind of father I wanta be now, and like I wanta turn time back and nobody can get old or die.

"I guess for a while my kid brother and me got along. We used to play show business when we were real small. I never thought of that before till the dream. And I never played show business with my Ronny. Somehow lately I've gotten around to callin' him 'my Ronny.' I never did that much before, either.

"But I wish I had done more with my kid, and maybe I'm sorry that me and my brother didn't get along better, too. My brother and my kid are often the same in my mind. I can see it in the dream.

"And my mother—I'm tellin' her I don't need her for my son or myself, and yet, maybe down deep, I'm so desperate I wish chicken soup would work on my son.

"I keep wantin' to go back like when I was small and my poor pop was alone, and I try to help him out, as if I could turn back time and start all over and be a kid myself—a really good kid, 'cause maybe I let my pop down, especially at the hospital when he was dyin'—my kid could be born again maybe or young again and all this—what's happenin' today—wouldn't be happenin', and my kid would be all the things I really want my kid to be, now." He rubbed his hands.

"But I know it ain't gonna happen. I'm in a daze like. And every once in a while I come out of it, and I start cryin' all over again.

"And my poor wife, she feels just like me, only she can hide it better. Only time will tell."

"It's been three years now, actually a little more, I been in therapy, and I'm still tryin' to just work things through, like you say. Going over it and over it again, all the time, and I'm doing fine. Everything is fine except my worryin' about my kid. I'll never stop worryin' till I know for sure if he's gonna make it. He's a cripple as it is. He isn't ready yet for an artificial leg, and when he walks on his crutches, he's all bent over like—like an old man. Looks like my pop when he was old, hunched over and walkin' with a limp and a cane, real slow. Every day I keep thinkin' about him and his cancer. But you say we still should try stoppin' anyway like we planned to see how things go? Sure, sure. I think I can and I know I can always phone for an appointment if I need you, especially with my boy so sick and all." He looked at me as if challenged. "But I still want to try it alone, like you said I should, even though I am a little scared—of what could happen to him—my kid."

After a month Harry and I agreed to interrupt formal therapy for a period of one-half year to see how Harry got along on his own.

In about six months Harry returned for one session. "Hello, Doctor. Let me tell you I been real good—but my boy . . ."

It's been more than one-half year, and he's doing well except for his realistic worry about his kid. I'd feel as lousy as he if it were my kid— maybe lousier. He works regularly, with only a rare twinge of anxiety now and then which he handles by reminding himself and analyzing himself.

Two more surgeries, the kid has had. It must mean the end is inevitable—six months, a year or two, sometimes longer, but soon. I remembered a seventeen-year-old girl I once saw on the autopsy table—a beautiful girl—she had an osteogenic sarcoma of her leg, also, with metastasis. Harry knows how sick his boy is. I can see in his eyes that he knows.

Harry, you're a brave guy. You've grown, as you wanted to. Part of you is dying and yet you're holding on "real good"—like you say. I could see you more often now in your crisis. Many psychiatrists would. But for you and your problem, it would be helpful, and a further step for you, if you could do it alone, without me, without a parent.

One spring two and a half years after we stopped therapy Harry phoned my secretary to make an appointment and had to wait several days to see me. "It's not an emergency," she quoted, "but he would like to see you as soon as he can."

Harry entered. His black eyes were sunken, and he looked thinner than I had ever seen him.

"Well," he began slowly. "My kid passed away. I told your secretary there was no emergency. When I called, we had already had the funeral a couple of days before. I thought of askin' you to come to the funeral. I thought you would of, but then I—I wanted to handle it myself to show myself I didn't need you, and I could handle it all alone, just like I been doin' with the rest of my life. So I decided not to ask you. But I didn't tell your secretary when I phone, 'cause I wanted to tell you myself." His dark eyes turned on me. They were disconsolate but not filled with the terror I had seen in them years before.

"My son's death that I watched happen before my eyes over the last year didn't throw me. Scared, yeah, but it didn't throw me—not like my father dyin'. I just am a different guy.

"But I ain't got no kid any more." He rested his head in his hands. "I came in to tell you, Doctor, 'cause I think of you as a friend, about my Ronny."

"I appreciate it, Harry. I feel as if I knew your boy." Harry saw the tears in my eyes.

"When I knew he wasn't gonna make it, I kept thinkin' of my whole life with my kid, and how different I wanted it to be—and how I wish I could've changed all the years with him and with my kid brother, too.

"And I remembered again my own father dyin' and how scared I was. But not with my kid. I wasn't too scared with him—watchin' him grow thin and pale and waste away in our home like an old man. I wasn't scared. I just felt bad—so bad for my kid. And finally we took him to the hospital, and I thought of my whole life again—in the past years, and I kept going over and over it again, what you and me talked about, Doctor, and the only wish I had was that my kid wasn't sick and I could start out all over with him bein' a little kid, so we could be friends as he was growin' up, just like that dream that I once told you about, Doctor. I've had dreams like it again, so many times. It's like tellin' good jokes. The best ones come up again and again with only a little twist here and there. . . ."

And so I hear from Harry occasionally, by phone, and once in a while he drops in to say hello. He's holding his own now, "real good"—the new Harry.

Chapter 6
Dannie the Cancer Patient

Dannie's tanned face was thin, worn, and serious. He sat down heavily in the chair across from me, his right hand over his lower abdomen. His surgeon, Dr. Rodney V. Johnson, had phoned me of the referral several days before.

"I was just operated on three months ago, doctor. I've got cancer, but I know I can lick it." He tried to smile despite the pain in his abdomen where the surgery had left him with a colostomy, a segment of bowel that opened through the abdominal wall from which excretion now took place. A section of the lower bowel where the malignancy was found near the rectum had been removed. His rectum was now permanently closed.

I knew my new patient's plight. "We tried to get as much of it as we could," Dr. Johnson had said on the phone, "but the regional lymph nodes were involved." His tone and choice of words betrayed his real knowledge of the prognosis. I knew, and Dr. Johnson was aware that I knew, that the widespread metastasis and extension from the original lesion left absolutely no hope that the surgery had cured the disease. "It's less than fifty-fifty," Dr. Johnson had said in answer to my questions. "But we want to offer him some hope."

"Yes," I agreed. "He must have some hope."

I used Dr. Johnson's carefully chosen words when Dannie saw me for the first time. "There is a chance for cure," I said. "I've spoken to your doctor at some length, and he said there is a chance." I lied even though I spoke the truth. And I hated it.

I was relieved that the patient helped me avoid dealing further with the question of his prognosis by assuming that he was cured. Thus, at our first meeting we established a misbegotten understanding that he had a normal lifespan ahead of him.

Still Dannie had his doubts. "I know that the healthier the mind, the healthier the body," Dannie said. "I think that if I'm perfectly well emotionally there would be no chance at all of the cancer growing again, and besides, everyone can use some psychiatry. I've got some problems with my family I've always wanted to straighten up."

At least he came to me at his own request. I had suspected that Dr. Johnson had referred him to me merely to relieve himself of a dying patient.

Patients who made it clear they dreaded the truth were told, "you have a little less than a fifty-fifty chance." Still some physicians believed that all patients should be told the truth no matter how painful. Such a mechanical approach made me shudder.

I recalled a consultation I had had years ago with a small, thin, tense man of fifty. The patient's internist had concealed the diagnosis from his patient. But the patient was sent to an X-ray doctor for irradiation treatment. When the patient asked why he was being treated, the radiologist said bluntly, "You have cancer of the stomach and you have just a few months left to live."

The cancer victim was speechless for a moment. Then he yelled at the radiologist, "You just killed me," and he slumped to the floor, burying his face in his hands as he wept and screamed.

During my consultation several weeks later, the patient sat in glum silence staring at my carpet. Suddenly he broke into frenzied sobs as if attending the funeral of a close loved one, and then just as suddenly returned to his withdrawn and silent state.

I recommended only the usual medical care plus nearly daily supportive psychotherapy by the referring internist, pointing out which drugs might be most useful for relief of his depression. I felt the family doctor would be able to render more useful psychotherapy than any psychiatrist, for the patient trusted him and shunned contact with any other physician after the radiologist's verdict of death. The patient, never clinically emotionally disturbed before this time, failed to recover from his shock. He died a year later of his malignancy, still in a state of frenzied torment.

And now Dannie, like the radiologist's patient, told me that he wished to avoid the pain of knowing that he was dying.

"Just before I got sick I was the healthiest guy alive," Dannie laughed at one of our early meetings. "I swam, played tennis, and ran track in college, and I still looked like a college kid, not like a man of thirty-four. I'm trying to figure out what I did wrong—maybe too much sex. I always was a ladies' man.' The dark shadows under his sunken eyes illuminated for a moment as he smiled. Then a grimace came over his face. "I keep getting these damned pains down here. They come and go all day and all night." He pressed his hand over his lower abdomen. "Excuse the gas," he said, as I smelled the flatus passing from his colostomy stump. "It's tough to be without an asshole. No muscle—what's it called?"

"The sphincter," I said.

"Yeah, that's what Dr. Johnson called it, so I can't control anything and my B.M.'s just come out into this little bag." He pointed to his abdomen. "But I keep it nice and clean. I change it a few times a day so there isn't much of a smell." His pale face with its even features and firm square jaw, once obviously full and strong, asked forgiveness with an apologetic smile.

"My wife is just great. She puts up with a lot even though she does complain once in a while. And my kids are wonderful. I've got three of them. My oldest kid is eight. She says she's going to be a nurse just to take care of me, and my little boy, Eddie, is five. He says, 'Daddy, I hope your bellyache is better today. I had a bellyache once, too, and it hurt so much.'" He laughed a grateful laugh. "It's nice to know they care."

Several weeks of our twice-weekly sessions had passed. "There's really been a helluva lot of pain lately, Dr. Sherwood." His lips were curled down, his eyes intense. "I know I'm getting better, though, 'cause the drainage from here is less." He touched his pants over his rectal area. "But the pain keeps me from sleeping. Florence gives me my shots whenever I ask for them, but that damned Demerol is so constipating, and I'm afraid I'll get hooked on it. So I take them only once or twice a day. I use Darvon instead. But I've been working every day at the store now even if it's just a couple of hours.

"I told you we have a pretty good business—furniture. We sell at five separate outlets with two or three salesmen at each plus the family spread out at the stores. This can be pretty rough, though working six or seven days a week. We're open Sundays too. My dad and my two brothers and I built up the business from nothing over the last twelve or fifteen years to where we all make a fairly good living and the business is still growing. And being a trained accountant helps, because as comptroller and vice-president I'm in charge of all of the finances.

"But that's what I wanted to talk about today—what happened once about a year ago. Damn! It's so hard to tell you this because I'm so ashamed of it." Tears came to his eyes. He pressed his hand to his abdomen. "I'd never done anything like it before. All of us work so hard at the business—me, my dad, my older brother, and my kid brother, though my dad takes it a little easier now, goes in only for six, seven hours a day and takes off Friday, Saturday, and Sunday unless it's Christmastime or something like that."

He smiled sadly. "I guess I really don't want to talk about what happened." His lips suddenly puckered. "His face quivered and screwed itself into folds and wrinkles like a boy who had just suffered some painful humiliation. Tears and mucous streamed down his face, which he wiped with a large embroidered handkerchief.

"Well, I've just got to tell you." He hesitated again. "I got the bookkeeper to make a few changes which she didn't understand, but she didn't question too much because she knows I'm a CPA. We never have an outside auditor like most businesses. I check the payroll and the income, and I supervise the inventory besides selling, too, when I have time. Well, this is what I did. About a year ago I took—I mean I—I really stole about eight thousand dollars. I covered it up by changing the inventory figures and nobody could ever find out. They all trusted me, and I swindled them." He sobbed. "My brothers and my dad trusted me and I did that to them. But I swore I'd put it back, especially after I got this thing," he pointed to his belly, "and first chance I get I'll put all of it back. I figured this is what I get for cheating."

He stopped, leaned forward on my desk, put his head down on his arm, covering his face, and wept again. "It sounds really silly, Dr. Sherwood, to believe this could happen to me because of what I did to my family, because I don't even believe in God or anything like that, and still I believe it did happen because I cheated. I've decided I'm going to tell them and give all the money back." He lifted his wet face. "I figure it's better really to come clean and tell them, even if I still get hold of enough money to sneak it all back without them knowing. Then I'll be forgiven and I'll—I'll get completely healed."

He was like a child who's been caught stealing from a trusting mother's purse. The punishment "decreed" by the fates came from his own conscience, a fact less absurd than what awaited him.

I felt myself cringing inwardly. Down deep he knew he was dying and he had to believe there was a way out. He fell back into a magical defense of his boyhood—that whenever he told the truth, his parents, or destiny, or some great power rewarded him, and that it would happen this time too, especially when his life was at stake.

I had learned from my patient that six years ago his family had been overwhelmed by grief. One of his mother's two brothers had died of bowel cancer at age forty-two. A familial tendency to develop bowel cancer existed in him and his kin. Dannie's parents probably were wary of his prognosis.

"We used the money to take a little vacation. Florence wanted to go to Spain, and she got a lot of clothes and jewelry for herself, and clothes for the kids, too, and some expensive rugs and drapes for the house. There wasn't much left of that eight thousand dollars. We told my folks we had saved money all these years just for a trip and we never even showed them the diamond earrings Flo brought back. Flo and I weren't getting along too well at that time, and I was under a lot of strain at work, too. The business needed to plow back all the money it could into new inventory, to expand, and to keep up with the growing competition. If you don't keep expanding in this business you get left behind. So there was nothing left for the big vacation pay we were hoping to get the last few years. Except for my parents, who draw a little more, we all get about fifteen thousand dollars a year— just enough to live on."

His bony face grew pale. "I was so scared I'd get caught because the cash position was already low. When my wife started talking about a divorce I fell to pieces. We'd been married nearly ten years and we hadn't had a real vacation since the trip we took to Mexico six or seven years ago when our two oldest kids were just babies." He paused.

"So there were some deep problems between you and your wife?" I said.

"Yeah. Don't ask me what kind, Doctor, because I don't know. I guess something bothered her. She said she was bored, disappointed in our marriage; I don't exactly remember what. I know her parents gave her everything she wanted. Maybe she expected more than I could give her. And you know," he said, raising his voice and looking up, "her parents never offered us one damned cent in all the years we've been married even though they could well afford to give us some money. I'll take that back. They bought new clothes for the kids once in a while, and Christmastime they bought the kids some toys, like a new bike for each of them last year. Our business was in rotten shape when we first got married. It almost went under and they never offered us a hint of a loan. And I never asked for one! Never!

"So last year Florence started complaining about no vacation and I told her we couldn't afford it. She really became bitter. She said she had worked hard enough for ten years, and she was getting older, and the business would always be there, and it was time we took a month-or-two vacation in Europe like everyone else. I wanted to go, too, but my brothers voted to invest all the surplus money in the business, like I said, so I had to go along with them.

"But things got worse at home. Florence and I were at each other's throats about everything, not just money. She kept saying my parents and brothers and the business were more important to me than she was, and there was no romance left in our marriage. That's when she started talking divorce. Sometimes she'd just get up and leave me and the kids and spend a few weekends away at her parents' house just to get away from the routine drudgery of being a housewife. And I'd get sore and tell her she was a prima donna, a damned spoiled rich kid who thought only about herself. Who else would leave three little kids to a Mexican maid who can't even speak English? And her parents agreed with me. They say they've spoiled her, too.

"Gee, Dr. Sherwood, without my wife and kids I've got nothing left—nothing—and I'm scared of being alone, especially now. But I know Florence really does love me. She tells me that she does all the time now, and I feel that we're really getting along good." He sank to one knee off his chair. "My butt hurts again so much," he groaned. "There's a deep aching there all the time and then come those sharp pains. It's the nerve endings, Dr. Johnson says. I guess it's trying to heal itself and grow back together in there, but the pain is killing me.

"By the way, Florence asked if she could meet with you. She says I've been coming now for a few months and she wants to meet you. And I think it's a good idea, because you'll get to know me better that way, through her eyes. I figure the better you know me, the more you can help me.

"So I'll tell you more about Florence and me, like you asked. Flo's the only one I've been able to talk with in my whole life. My mom just never talked with us boys except 'What do you want for supper?' and 'Did you do your homework?' She's not a bad person, but she never really talked with us, and if something bothered her she kept it to herself, always. And if something bothered me she just couldn't talk about it either. She's never even mentioned my being sick, never to this moment, and my pop is even worse. Business is the only thing he ever thought of in his whole life, the business and keeping us kids from tearing the house apart. He could really get sore if we started fighting. Otherwise he just never paid much attention to us except for school.

"And my brothers and I—we never got along, like I said. So Flo's been the first person in my life I could really talk with. Even though we fight a lot we've been able to talk about ourselves and the kids, and we've been pretty close ever since we got married—very close, in fact. We can really let our hair down to each other, and we know each other pretty good, I'd say, after about ten years of married life . . ."

Florence gazed sharply through green-blue eyes. She had an attractive face with a slightly aquiline nose. She was slender in a yellow knit dress, carefully chosen to accentuate the color of her eyes. She walked with sensual movements, like a woman cognizant of the impression she made upon onlookers. But there was a harshness in her voice that detracted from her, or perhaps the content of her message influenced how she sounded to me more than I was aware.

"I guess you know about some of the troubles Dannie and I have had," she said in a nasal tone. She lit a cigarette. "We almost separated before he got sick. I guess he told you that, too."

I nodded.

"I don't know what I'm going to do now," she said. "You see, I decided I wanted a divorce just about the time he got sick. We've been fighting since the day we got married eleven and a half years ago. I wasn't sure I wanted to get married then, but he really put on a campaign for me and I finally gave in."

Smoke sifted through her nostrils. "He lied to me about his family—how big their business was, and how prominent they were in the community, and about what he had, and about everything else. He led me to believe he owned a big part of the family business when his father really owned all of it. When we got married, he drove a Jaguar and he couldn't even afford a Chevy. For the last few months he's been asking me a dozen times a day if I love him. I always say, 'Yes,' because he's sick, but I don't, and I think I never really did. Now I don't know what to do about us.

"My mother used to tell me how poor she was when she was a kid growing up in Boston and how much she hated being poor. She got stuck in a miserable marriage to my father just because he had a little money. But all their lives she had nothing in common with him except me. She says he did nothing but work all the time, and he was always cold and unaffectionate toward her. So she decided not to have any more kids after me. I grew up alone, swearing I'd never marry a man I didn't really love just for security the way she did. And then I went ahead and did it anyway. I guess my mother's feelings took hold of me, despite myself. So I married a man who pretended to be well off when he really had almost nothing. I was a fool.

"Not long after I was born, times grew bad. My father lost almost everything he had in his real estate business and he had to go to work in a factory. My mother's nightmare came true. And so has mine."

She stopped, then suddenly spoke again as if remembering. "Did he tell you about the money, the money he took for our vacation?"

"Yes, he did. It was very hard for him to talk about it."

"Don't feel too bad," she said, "for his brothers, I mean. Dannie has the brains. He's the accountant, the only one who finished college. He does all the thinking and all the managing and all the worrying, and still his brothers get paid just as much, or just as little, I should say. That's the way their father wants it. He's a tightwad, a crotchety old man. I know he owns the business, but it's Dannie who spends day and night looking after the stores. He stays till they close at seven o'clock, long after most of the help and both his brothers have gone home. That's why he's never had time for me or the kids.

"So he took a bonus. He deserves it. It wasn't that much anyway, and now he feels he's got to tell them. It will embarrass both of us. There's no reason for him to tell. They might even think I put him up to it, even though we deserved the extra money. But Dannie has a feeling a confession will help him. I don't see how. Dr. Johnson told the family privately what Dannie's chances really are, and I feel sorry for him, and I'm trying to be kind to him, but confessing won't help him live longer, and I just don't think he should tell." She lit another cigarette and smoked it slowly. "I probably won't try to get a divorce now, anyway. I'll just wait and see, for a while at least."

The next day Dannie, serious-faced, sat opposite me. "I was always kind of mean to my little brother, and I was a kind of smart-alecky kid," he said, confessing his sins further.

"Both my brothers always thought I was the one my parents liked best because I was good in school and they were lousy. 'The favorite son,' they would say to me. Once I called my little brother a dunce-head when he failed a couple of subjects in the eighth grade. My older brother spoke up and told me to shut up and not think I was so smart all the time, and he was right. We got into a big fight and pounded hell out of each other till my mom and dad got home from the store. We had only one store then. My dad sent my older brother to his room and took away his allowance for a month, and I was just as much to blame as he was. But I guess I was always favored because I was the good student. It was really a dirty trick on my brother to let him take the whole blame.

"I was the favorite all the way through college, too. My big brother went for a year or two, then he dropped out. My kid brother didn't even want to start college, he hated school so much. So I got to go while they worked in the stores. And they teased me day and night, they were so jealous. And I deserved their teasing. They were working and I wasn't. But my dad always promised to pay for anyone who wanted to go through school. I'm glad to say once I started working in the stores we all got equal salaries—except for what I took. Pop always said when he dies his sons would all get an equal one-third share each, so we wouldn't fight among ourselves, and we haven't had any serious fights for years now. Maybe I still thought I should be the favorite son, and that's why I took the extra money. That was a dumb thing to think."

He paused suddenly. He had been avoiding other thoughts. "Florence asked me not to tell, Dr. Sherwood. She asked me not to say anything to my dad and brothers about the money. It will make us look terrible, she says. But I told her I felt I just have to tell them, and then she really got sore at me. I don't want her to be mad at me now, especially when I'm beginning to lick this thing. And when I got well—I mean completely healed—Flo and I are going to give one really big party, and my brothers and their families and every one of our friends will be there, and the champagne is going to flow all over the place, and we'll have one helluva time." He smiled. "And you'll be there, too, won't you, Doc?"

The question seemed innocent enough. It was the answer that I feared. He wanted a promise—a promise of life for him, and what would I, the physician, be if I promised and my promise was a sham? I'd thought it over a thousand times. He doesn't really want the truth. So I'd play the game, and he'd play the game, and someday the game would out.

"I'd like very much to be there, Dannie, very much. And if fighting helps, you're the kind of guy who will be able to give a party like that."

I felt his desperation and my sense of helplessness and his need to bolster me if only to bolster himself. If he could get me to believe he would live, I'd convince him he would live, and his denial fostered by mine would grow stronger and he'd continue to live and work and be part of life and save us both from reality, with its terror and depression and frenzy and hopeless pain. And he'd chatter good-naturedly and laugh and laugh and tell jokes and laugh, and I'd laugh too, until the day that his obdurate malignancy enlarged and spread with an ugly tenacity that refused to shrink away despite the chemotherapy and X-ray treatments that I knew would probably be tried in the near future.

Why in hell had I taken him on, knowing he would be tortured until the moment of his death? Didn't I know how painful living with him would become? I think of him at times in bed at night before I fall asleep, and when I awaken in the middle of the night to the ticking of the clock, and when I first open my eyes in the morning, and when I have a few minutes of quiet sitting in my office looking out the window, and while I eat my lunch, and while I walk to the toilet, or stroll down the street, or go anywhere. Again and again and again I think of him, and my anger against death arises—anger is my defense—rationalized by the thoughts that such deaths could be avoided. If just a few of the many billions of dollars squandered on wars were put to proper use, more questions about malignancies would be answered. And now I wish I had gone into the more fruitful field of pathology and cancer research. At this moment I would be faced with a neutral, peaceful microscope trained on a glass slide with a few pink-and-purple-stained aberrant cells swirling in a sea of colored glass, not the living, weeping, pained, dying Dannie whom I hate at this moment, hate because of my fear and my helplessness at his coming death and at my own.

A few more weeks of sessions had passed. Dannie came in one day and said, "I don't know, Doctor. I'm having trouble sleeping now. The pain is always there in my butt and here in front too." He sank down on his knees off his chair. "This is the way I sit sometimes, kneeling. It's a good position to be in, too, in case I want to pray." He forced the pain from his face with a facsimile of a smile, but the pain quickly sprang back, then after a few moments diminished again.

"My wife is still quarreling with me. She insists it won't be very beneficial if I tell my dad and my brother, but I keep thinking it would be good for me to tell them. I mean, I—don't believe in God—or anything like that, but I've a strange feeling, like I told you before, that if I come clean with them, this thing," he indicated with his thumb, "is more likely to go away. It's getting better, anyway, because yesterday and the day before, even though it hurt a little more, I could sleep with only two shots of Demerol at night. The week before I needed a third shot, but I promised myself I wouldn't give in to the pain, and I decided to limit myself to two shots a night, no matter what. Because I figure if I take more than two shots it's getting worse, not better."

He groaned. "Sometimes, though, it's just unbearable, but I know I have got to be careful not to get addicted because it's tough to get out of addiction, isn't it?" He turned to look at me.

"Yes," I nodded, "but if you need it, Dannie—"

"I really don't. And I'm not giving in to this thing no matter what. Besides, that Demerol is so constipating. That and my colostomy cause me to have such hard B.M.'s I lose more water through my colostomy than people with a normal bowel do, Dr. Johnson said, so I get real dry inside. I have to take those damned enemas every day and I spend most of the morning sitting on the toilet just trying to get those rocks out of me. When I do, I feel better. I know I'm getting well.

"My bottom heals a little every time I lie in the sunlight and let the air in, so I spend three or four hours just lounging outside every afternoon baking my bare ass. I can tell it's getting better because the drainage is less, or at least it's not worse, and if it doesn't get worse it means it has to be getting better. But why it all takes so fuckin' long beats me! It's been nearly a year, hasn't it, since my surgery?

"Jesus! I spend most of the day just taking care of myself. I hardly get to the office any longer. We had to hire another comptroller full time to help me, so I just supervise him when I get a chance. I don't know what they're going to do with him when I get back full time, but that'll be his worry, because I told them I expect to be back within the next six months."

I listened to Dannie, struggling against death. And I felt a terrible anguish in myself. I listened to his denial, his self-protective, adaptive-defensive struggle against death, and I thought of what I'd feel like if I were he, and for a moment I became Dannie and it was too much—too damned much to take, and part of me wanted to run away from him, from his pain and from mine.

Dannie's bargaining for life was different from that of most victims, who try to make a deal with God or fate in order to live a bit longer. Dannie's bargaining was in the form of a confession to be followed by a hoped-for forgiveness and reprieve from death. He struggled tirelessly. The act of battling itself was vital to him.

Again I pondered, how much had my dread of death interfered with my treatment of Dannie? An anguish took hold of me. Some patients should be told the truth. Others beg to avoid it. Should they be told anyway? And if told would they suffer from the truth as the radiologist's patient of long ago had? Or had I allowed my own fear of death, my childhood trepidation, my own unwillingness to face death, my identification with Dannie to overrule that which was best for him?

Some memories of my childhood came to me, of a neighbor, Mr. Joe, whom I loved when I was five. I remember him walking down the street toward me, smiling, with an ice cream cone in his hand, as he often did in the evening on his way home from work. Unexpectedly he slumped to the ground, clutching his chest. The ice cream went splattering to the sidewalk. Another neighbor ran to pick him up. When he turned Mr. Joe over, I saw Mr. Joe's pale and bloodless face, while a small stray dog began licking the ice cream that was intended for me. I ran into my house crying as people carried him away. I never saw him again, and I never forgot the look on his face as he was dying.

Two years later my grandmother died. My mother's sobbing touched me deeply. The cold fall winds rattled the stiff, brown leaves around my grandmother's grave site as her casket was lowered into the ground before my eyes. I was terrified that she would be suffocated when I saw the male relatives shoveling the dirt over her casket.

Next came my observations of the dying during World War II and after that during my medical experiences. I knew that my fear of death and my wish to master and control the fear had been one of my reasons for going into medicine—to gain the imagined power of the physician, the controller of life and death.

Patients had died while I was examining them, even while I spoke with them, but I was always able to limit my thoughts of death, to allow the forces of repression to take over by preoccupying myself with necessary medical chores. Never before had I had to deal with death so intimately as I did with Dannie, as I observed his face day after day growing waxen and tormented, the human behind it so demanding, so pleading, so depending upon me for succor and solace, for hope and cure.

Now Dannie knelt down in pain, and I wished him dead. The torment was too great—for me. I wanted to save myself from the gnawing expectation he had of me to cure him, not merely to save him from further pain. I felt ashamed. It was Dannie's pain that made me feel so troubled, but it was for my sake, not for Dannie's, that I wished him dead.

"I love you, Abe," he said as he knelt. I was startled to hear him say this, yet pleased that he felt comfortable enough to say it to me. He stood up and put his arms around me, and I put mine around him. He was crying. Tears threatened to break my composure, too, even though I knew it was all right to cry. I heard myself say in a stilted voice, "I love you too, Dannie. You're a brave guy. You deserve to make it." And for a moment I, too, fell into Dannie's childlike, guilt-laden, magical, wishful attitude. I felt that his few misdeeds, stealing and cheating, little deserved what fate had inflicted on him. At the same time I knew that his cancer was no punishment, and that our penitence would provide no dispensation for him.

At the moment of the hug I realized Dannie's unconscious had read my wish, and he was comforting me for it. He saw my anguish and my ambivalence toward his tortured life, and he forgave me. He realized in that flash that he and I both knew that he would die, and that I was pained by it, and that I wanted to ease my pain even at his expense. He had slipped into my feelings, as I had into his.

Throughout our work, objective interpretations had been minimal. Respecting him and understanding and reacting to his needs were my prime methods of psychotherapy.

I did acknowledge, with Dannie's agreement, the significance to him of winning and retaining a beautiful wife like Florence. Originally, her sexual attractiveness had once again allowed him to triumph over his two brothers. She made him feel important. I probed no further.

From time to time I phoned him in the evening to see how he was, or just to say hello. I constantly wondered if he should be told, told what he already suspected. From the start, I had collaborated with Dr. Johnson in his medication. Now I actually prescribed the narcotics, tranquilizers, and sleeping pills, carefully adjusting the dosage after phone consultations with Dr. Johnson, who saw Dannie once or twice a week. There was a practicality to this collaboration. I saw Dannie frequently and knew most about his pain and anxiety.

"Don't hesitate to take more pain-killer if you need it, Dannie," I said.

Dannie replied. "Like I was saying, two Demerols at night is all I'll let myself have, and I don't need morphine prescriptions any more. I just won't take any."

Two days later we began another session.

"She's such a good wife," Dannie began. "She takes care of me fourteen hours a day. And she drives me to all my doctors and everywhere else I have to go. Now Dr. Johnson wants me to get X-ray treatments every day for the next six weeks, so I have to go to still another doctor, plus getting physiotherapy for my back pain. I could hardly get here today. But I still want to continue our twice-a-week sessions, and maybe increase them to three or four times a week, if you have time. It's the only way to get cured."

His face remained serious. "The pain won't let up now. It keeps nagging at me, and I'm bloated all the time. But I know that's what happens when you're healing. Once I broke my arm playing baseball when I was a kid. I tripped when I slid into the second baseman stretching a hit. I was safe." He tried to smile. "But my arm hurt for months even when it was almost healed. My backside is still raw, though I'm in the sun every day, but that's getting better too. It's almost a year now, and I know if I've made it to here, I've made it for good." He paused. A look of gratitude relieved the tension in his face.

"Now I've got to tell you. Yesterday I told my parents and my brothers what I did."

He sounded bizarrely dramatic to me, a man near death, still preoccupied with a triviality of the living.

"It was really tough to tell them. I had a vision of my dad yelling and telling me what a rotten son I was, and my big brother taking a punch at me, and my mother falling to pieces. And you know, they surprised me. They just listened. My father turned pale and didn't say anything for a while, and my mother just stood there. I knew she couldn't talk either."

Dannie's eyes grew moist, but no tears came, only a slight smile of relief. "Finally my dad said he understood and to forget it, to pay them back over the next few years. It felt so good to tell them and I'm glad I did, except for one thing. The night before I told them, Flo again made me give my solemn promise not to say anything. She made me swear I wouldn't, and then I went ahead and told them anyway." A sadness took over his face. "I just had to tell them; I had to." His face suddenly puckered dolefully. He looked like a small, thin boy as he began to cry openly. "I just had to.

"And my dad said no matter what, the business was one-third mine just like they always promised. It goes to me and my family when my folks pass away, no matter what happens, even though there's no written agreement between us. We're a close family and everything belongs to the kids when the parents go. That's what my mother and dad both said. Flo wanted me to make sure of this, and that's another reason she gave when she said not to tell them, because she's afraid my dad might change his mind someday and leave it all to my brothers, but I know he won't. He's not that kind of guy, even though he could get pretty angry and rough at times with us when we were kids when we did something wrong. He was shocked when I told him, but he forgave me. And my mother and brothers, they joined in and were nice, even though my brothers said nothing at first. But my mom made them promise to listen to her and dad and not to fight over the business after my parents are gone.

"And, God, I'm so glad I told them, so glad." He rubbed his abdomen. "So glad. Then they began to say it was probably Flo's idea anyway, and they understood the pressure I was under. They never did like Flo, and they always said she was only interested in money. I told them it wasn't true. It was my idea to 'borrow' the money. That's how I put it. I really only 'borrowed' it, and someday I was going to pay it all back, every nickel of it."

He suddenly became breathless.

"Ooh, the pain! It's killing me." He stood up from his chair and bent over with both hands on his mid-abdomen. "It's been rough today, but I had to come to see you so I—I could tell you what I did— and I'm so glad." The pain let up.

"But I wish you'd speak to Flo again, would you? I know I can trust you not to tell her. It's so important to me that she not find out I told. I want you to see her because she's been pretty tough on me lately— edgy and tense, and she's always screaming at me and the kids. Her life's been hell too since I got sick. Sometimes I don't know what to do to please her. I know we never go anywhere any more, except to my doctors, because of this thing. Still she does go out alone regularly to her girl friends' to play bridge or to a movie. I never feel like going with her—the damned drainage from my bottom, my colostomy smells worse, the constipation is getting so bad, like I told you, and the pain. . . . While my stomach—bowel, I guess I should say—is healing, the pain is getting stronger." He tried to smile. "I think I bellyache too much about my aching belly.

"I don't know. Maybe she's so tense because we haven't had sex in such a long time. A few months after my operation I just lost interest in sex—could hardly get one up so I would set her off with my finger or go down on her just to satisfy her, but for nearly a year now she hasn't wanted even that any more. Says she really doesn't like it that way and would rather wait till I'm feeling better. So she doesn't have any kind of a sexual outlet now. Make her understand, Abe, she's got to be patient till I get better. She trusts you and says she wants to see you again, anyway.

"By the way, I've been losing my appetite of late, too, something that never happened before. . . ."

A few days later Florence phoned for an appointment and came alone to my office.

"I think he told them," Florence began. She puffed again on a cigarette, smoke drifting upward and circling her stern, green-eyed face. A deep redness of her eyes and the skin surrounding her eyes and nose reflected her many days of weeping. "I'm not sure, but I got that feeling when I saw his brothers last night. They came over to see Dannie.

"I'll bet you know," she said, looking up at me unflinchingly. She read my expressionless face correctly. There would be no reply. "But it doesn't matter, now. I've had it with all of them—Dannie's whole family. They've always been nasty to me. His older brother even hinted that if something happens to Dannie, Dannie's third would remain in their family. I thought to myself, 'Damn you, I'll start a lawsuit if Dannie's share isn't given to me and the kids.' But there is no written partnership agreement, and the whole rotten business legally all belongs to the parents, even though Dannie's worked so hard ever since we were married to build it up. We deserve our third.

"I'm hoping his parents will give us our share for their grandchildren's sake. Dannie never believed much in life insurance, and all we have is a small policy the business bought for each so-called partner. I'd hate to ask my parents to help out. They don't have much and they've always given us what they could. Dannie's hospital and doctor bills have wiped out most of our savings even though we have hospitalization insurance, and his parents have continued Dannie's salary. I just cashed in our last one-hundred-dollar government bond, one we got for a wedding gift."

She paused and said in a dry voice, "Our wedding. It should never have taken place." Her thin lips were tight as she spoke. "I guess I can get a job selling dresses at Saks where I used to buy my clothes." Her face became more taut.

"It's been too much for me and the kids—just too much. I can't take it any longer, Dr. Sherwood," she said hoarsely. "It's just too much, watching him waste away like this. He keeps waking me up all through the night to give him shots for pain and to talk with him half the night while he cries. And he begs me to tell him again and again that I care about him and that I love him. All night long he keeps asking me, and I keep telling him I do.

"I finally decided to ask him to sleep alone in our bedroom because he's always tossing and groaning except for an hour or two after I give him the Demerol, and there's just no sleep for either of us. I've had to move our son into the bedroom with our youngest daughter, and I sleep with the older one now." She dropped her head in her hands for a moment, and spoke slowly. "I told you how I feel about Dannie. It's been hard on me too, very hard."

She turned and looked fully at me again. "I'll bet you think I'm hateful because I'm not in love with Dannie and he's dying—and I'm selfish because I think so much of what's going to happen to me and the kids afterwards."

I hesitated. I felt her coldness toward Dannie, though she did all she could be expected to do for him and more than many wives would. She had even administered some of the enemas to his colostomy when he found it difficult in the last few weeks. Did I dislike her? Yes, to some degree, but could I condemn her for her failure to love Dannie?

"Flo, you've done more than your duty in caring for him. Nobody can demand that you be in love with Dannie."

She seemed startled when I called her by her first name, though I had done so before. Her face lit up slightly and her clenched jaws relaxed. She seemed assured against an expected attack from me, though she detected accurately my sorrow for Dannie and my resentment toward her for her failure to love him as he needed to be loved now.

How would I feel if I were dying and had a wife who hated me and detested our years together? What chance was there to make amends or to start another life? If I had given everything I knew how to give, enslaved by my need for a wife like Florence, how could I not hate her? And then I grew angry at Dannie for being so dumb as to blind himself and sell himself to as narcissistic and selfish—though beautiful—a woman as Florence. Her rapacious demands would always be beyond him. I hated her, doubly, for both Dannie and myself. These were moments, painful seconds, when I grew nearly indistinguishable from my patient.

Yet all the time that I felt these things, I still knew that I was not, nor ever would be, Dannie, and that there was more to their problems than just Dannie's point of view. I remembered that more than once I had been convinced of the righteousness of an earnest wife or husband, only to be flabbergasted a few days later by the contradictory and equally convincing arguments of the mate.

Flo had her needs, too, and most of all she needed a supportive ally to help her with her ordeal.

"No one can demand that you love him, Flo," I repeated. "And as for thinking about yourself, you must plan for what will come after Dannie passes away. How could you not think of yourself?"

She was relieved by my confrontation. I, as an authority figure, an unconscious parental surrogate, had lessened her guilt.

She let go of the armrest that she had been clutching with both hands and settled back in her chair.

"I want to tell you something else, Dr. Sherwood," she said. "I've been feeling very uneasy for many months. I've been thinking of discussing something with someone all that time. I couldn't tell anyone, not even my best girl friend. I wanted to talk with a psychiatrist too." She stopped once more. She looked hurt as her reddened face flushed deeper. Then she gasped, struggling against a strong urge to cry again.

"I've got to tell because I—I feel dirty, somehow, and I want you to know. All these past months when Dannie thought I was out playing cards with the girls, I've been seeing someone—an old schoolmate of Dannie's whom Dannie and I used to double-date with when they were students at USC. This fellow and his wife were separated a year or so ago, and he called to visit Dannie in the hospital after Dannie's operation. A few months later he called me again to say hello and ask about Dannie. I let him know that Dannie was dying but didn't know it. We got together once or twice for lunch and we talked—about Dannie, and then about ourselves and our marriages. I've always admired Graham. He's a person of class. He told me that he enjoyed our company, though he and Marge, that's his wife, got together with us only once in a while after Dannie and I were married.

"Graham is an executive with an international banking firm, and he's away from home a lot. He deals with important people from all over the world. Graham and Marge started finding out how different they were right after they were married. She never liked to leave home to travel with him, though he'd asked her to many times. I think that would be a terribly exciting kind of life. He thought he was sure after twelve years of married life they were just not for each other and so he moved out and has his own apartment now. He left Marge with the two kids.

"But it's all so very complicated. Graham and I fell in love with each other, and we've been having an affair for nearly—what is it?— over a year—a crazy kind of a fling. Now he's in a turmoil about whether or not to get a divorce. He says he really loves me, but the divorce thing has gotten to him because he wants his kids, too. He can't leave them, and his wife's screaming she wants him back."

Her voice broke into a high-pitched squeal as she began to cry. "And I've been going crazy over all of this for the last year and a half—Dannie with his operation and his pain, and his crying, and his bleeding, and his shots, and his toilet problems, and his smelly discharge, and running back and forth to all kinds of doctors with him all day long these last few months while he's getting worse, and the kids constantly tearing at me with no help in the house, and Graham and his hangup about divorcing—and what am I really going to do after Dannie goes? It's just too much for me to take, that's all—just too Goddamn much." She continued crying. "I can't take it any more, I just can't. I've got to talk with you—or someone—I'm sick too."

After a few moments of weeping she broke off. Her voice was quiet now. "Oh, I almost forgot. Dannie asked if you'd come out to see him at home. He can't keep his appointment tomorrow. He's got too much pain. Pain. Pain. That's all I've heard for a year now." Her voice rose rapidly into a frenzy again. "Pain. Pain. Pain. Damn it. I hate him," she shrieked. "I hate him. He's a mess of rotting cancer inside his body. He's filthy with cancer, and he's dying right next to me in bed, and when I touch him, I feel sick, and when I smell him and all the shit that comes out of him, I hate it, and I hate him, and I ask, 'Why did it have to happen to me?' I can't help it. I just can't help it. I hate him!"

She stopped suddenly in frozen silence, a look of pallid horror on her face, as if something had escaped her lips that should have remained secret. She looked up and said quietly, "And I'll bet you really hate me now, too."

I was stunned—stunned not by her words, but by the strength of her feelings. She had to say it. She had spoken her feelings irretrievably, and now she expected me to be outraged at her hatred for Dannie.

"No, Flo." I shook my head. "I don't hate you—not at all. Maybe we'd all feel the way you do without knowing it."

Now it became clear to me why she felt so strong in her disgust for Dannie. The horror of his illness had become magnified by her unconscious predisposition to feel trapped by a certain type of man. Graham represented the fantasy by which she could escape this fate. Her mother felt imprisoned by a disappointing marriage. Flo, fearing in her childhood daydreams that she would be equally unhappy, had always been precipitously ready to act out her mother's impulses to escape an unhappy married life, even before Dannie's illness.

I let Flo feel that her words were acceptable by making no further allusion to them.

"You were telling me, Flo, that Dannie couldn't make it to my office and you wanted me to make a house call?"

She answered in a whisper. "He said you promised you'd find time in the evening, like you did a couple of weeks ago."

"Yes, I'll arrange to come out in the evening. I'll phone first."

Flo's guilt over her affair as well as her overwhelming conflicts over Dannie moved her to tell me about Graham. In her unconscious, I was the parental authority from whom she must gain solace and exoneration for her deeds. But did she know that I usually discussed with my patients any information given to me by family members while keeping private from the family any confidential material imparted to me by my patient? Of course she did. That was it. An additional unconscious dynamic motivated her to "confess" to me. She knew that I would make an exception, that I would refrain from informing Dannie of her affair. Her secret would be my secret. By my failure to inform Dannie she would gain more than just "parental" permission. I would become an accomplice.

There would be only sorrow for Dannie if I were to inform him. Nor would my silence be a violation of the confidentiality afforded Dannie, for at this moment Florence, too, was a patient.

I said nothing to Florence, though I felt her unconscious was reading my thoughts. If I said anything, she would feel that I was critical of her. Her gratitude was expressed in her reply to my next words.

"Flo, Dannie hasn't long to go."

"I won't leave him," she said. "You don't have to worry about that. I have feelings for Dannie too.

"But I feel 'dirty' somehow, and I needed to talk with you about it."

"Our time is almost over, Flo. Let's set up another meeting or two and go on."

"Yes, whenever you have time."

"Dannie and I—we've never had much of a real marriage," Flo said. "He seems to want to think so, now that this has happened. But all we've ever had have been small talk and fights about money and in-laws. He thinks my parents are stingy, that they have money stashed away and should help us out now that we need it. I'm an only child so my parents have always given me everything that they could, and I've learned to like nice things. And why shouldn't I?

"My dad never made much of himself, though he's always tried in his own way. My parents even still pretend to their friends that he's an executive high up at Lockheed, but the highest he's ever been is assistant purchasing engineer. And he isn't even an engineer. He's really just a clerk with a big title and no pay to go with it. He's been there twenty-seven years, and my mother and dad spend every cent of his salary pretending they're rich. They owe half-a-dozen stores in town. A few years ago they even had some furniture repossessed because they couldn't find any bank to lend them the money, their credit was so bad. And my mother was frightened to death her friends would find out about it.

"Every once in a while they become terrified that my dad will be laid off, like last year when Lockheed lost that big contract to Boeing. You probably read about it in the papers. He was glad to take a big cut in salary just to hang on to his job. So my mother always kept pushing me to marry rich: 'Find a nice guy with money and marry him.' And when Dannie came along, she fell in love with him because he was good-looking and she thought he had money, and so I married him—probably for her, not for me. And then he became a big disappointment to her just like my dad is.

"There were lots of men interested in me. But I thought a college graduate knew everything because I only finished high school. That's why I married Dannie, and then I found out how dull an accountant could be. Even with his degree he doesn't know very much except, maybe, about business. And when I tell my mother why I married Dannie she says to me, 'It was your choice, not mine, so live with it.' Sometimes I hate her! I never could tell her anything. All she had in mind was for me to marry a rich guy so she could look good, because her own marriage was such a big flop. 'Your father knows nothing about the better things in life. All he knows about is tools and parts for airplanes and not much of that.

"That's what I heard when I was a kid—lots of bitter quarrels between them about money and about what my dad should have done and what he shouldn't have done and how dull and stupid he was and how he couldn't make a decision without his family butting in, and how they never go anywhere or do anything because my dad just likes to stay home, and he only thinks of her as a maid to clean the house and carry out the garbage. And he says she doesn't understand how hard he works, and how worried and tired he is all the time, and that she's just selfish.

"Whenever she wanted to break up the marriage and leave him, he'd start to cry and she'd come back, not just because she felt sorry for him, but most of all because she didn't want to bring up a daughter without a father. That was what my childhood was all about—that and how my mother could have married this man or that man who's now worth plenty as a big-time lawyer or businessman, and how disappointed she's been all her life married to a meek guy who can never get promoted because he didn't go to school, and because he's afraid he's not smart enough to learn something new, and because he's too scared to push himself with his boss.

"So I made up my mind I would never have the same dull life she has, skimping on this and that so she can buy a ring or bracelet to pretend to her friends they're well off. They keep the fact that they're still in hock a pretty good secret—but not from me.

"And my dad. He's a frightened, bitter guy who knows he's a failure. He just keeps to himself. 'Hello' and 'goodbye' and a few words in between is all he ever said to me. We could never talk about anything.

"So finally after all these years I got to know a guy like Graham who has real class and charm. The kind of man I've always wanted, and I fell for him in a big way. It wasn't that Dannie was sick. Graham came along at a time in my life when I knew I couldn't stay married any longer anyway.

"Our marriage was no good from the beginning. But then the kids started coming and you know the old story, Dr. Sherwood. Most wives stick it out, but not me. I wasn't going to make the same mistake my mother did. I decided, 'I've only got one life and I might as well live it with the right person.' So I made my decision even before Dannie got sick. Then, one day by chance, Graham phoned about Dannie. It just kind of happened. We got to know each other, and I became closer to Graham than I have to anyone in my whole life. It didn't take place just because he was separated and lonely and I was lonely too. Graham is just the kind of exciting man I've always wanted to meet."

I saw Dannie two days after my second meeting with Florence and I continued to make visits to Dannie's home once or twice a week. By the third week he was unable to arise from his bed. He began vomiting continually, making it necessary to supplement his diet with intravenous feedings and to hire a full-time day nurse. Dannie's skin had become jaundiced, his eyes deeply sunken and weary.

As I entered his bedroom one day, he fought to sit up. His usual, though frequently forced, thin smile of greeting was absent. His jaundice told me his liver was probably involved in an obstructive type of metastasis from his bowel cancer. The end could not be far off.

"Hello, Dannie." I heard myself say.

"Hi, Abe," he answered feebly. Then he looked down at his bloated abdomen and said, "It just won't let up any more, Abe. It won't stop. I've been fighting it and fighting it, but the pain won't let up. Dr. Johnson has me come to the hospital every morning now for the cobalt treatment and chemical injections—Cytoxan, is that what you call it? The nurse and Flo practically have to carry me. Dr. Johnson wants me back in the hospital, but I told him I didn't want to go." His face was a fixture of grief and pain. "This is where I want to be, right here at home, in my own home, in my own bed. I'll go to the hospital for the treatment every day if I have to, but this is where I stay." He waved his hand around the room. "I'm not leaving here no matter what."

He was clinging to life. He was 'aware' of what the hospital meant now. His denial was growing thin. I read it in his face.

"I had a shot of morphine an hour or two ago and it's beginning to hurt again. Even morphine won't stop it now." Weakness faded his voice into a whisper.

He began to cry. "It's been over a year and a half. I thought I had it licked, but some of the cells got away, Dr. Johnson explained. That's why they've started the Cytoxan and cobalt. They're trying to get those little cells that got away in my belly—those fuckin' little cells that can kill you!" He held his index finger close to his thumb like pincers. "Those little tiny cells that got away—and all the time I was beating the cancer. I'd be all better except for those few cells that won't disappear and keep growing in my belly."

Reality momentarily tore away his shredded defenses.

His voice rose. "Is this the way it's going to be? Is this how it happens? I feel like screaming and crying, 'God help me; someone help me; don't let me slip away like this. For God's sake, grab me.' Abe, don't let me slip away. Abe, Abe, I thought we had this thing licked! All the time I thought we had it licked! Oh no, don't let me die. Someone, God, someone help me! There must be some answer. Look, I'm alive and breathing, someone help me, grab me, help me, hold my hand, Abe."

I reached out and took his outstretched hand. Drops of sweat rolled down his forehead and coalesced with his tears as they fell on the bed.

"Oh, Abe, there must be a way," he gasped, short of breath and exhausted. "Some way! Maybe the cobalt, or the Cytoxan injections. They might get the cells. Jesus!" His voice lowered. "At least I've got my family here. Flo's in the next room, and she's right here when I want her. Sometimes I wake up in the middle of the night alone, and I realize what's really happening to me, and I'm so glad Flo's my wife. She's been so good to me. She loves me and she sticks by me and it's so much easier for me this way. I think of Flo, and the kids playing and laughing in the yard and the warm sunshine on the patio near the flowers and the people all around us in the neighborhood talking, and our friends, and I know I can't leave—I just can't and I won't. I tell you I won't leave and no cancer is going to make me." He continued weeping in exhausted fits, burying his face in the bedsheets.

Was he thinking that I had failed him? At that moment I felt as if I had. I realized that some part of me had begun to believe that I might be able to heal him, some omnipotent part of me that would save me from his horrible fate if I ever should develop the same disease. Strange that I could feel the most penetrating sorrow for him and resentment, both at the same time. Dannie had exposed my mortality to me.

And when he died, did I expect him to die without a whimper, "like a man"? Was it because I expected that of myself, demanded it of myself, yet feared that when my time came, I would flail myself and weep the way Dannie did? Was that why I felt so pained at this moment? Selfish that I should think of that now—think of myself rather than of him. He believed that the mind could heal a sick body—a promise I never made. But I did not disillusion him of that hope, either.

Should he have been informed despite his wish? Would the end now close at hand have been easier? Or would the certain knowledge of his death have "killed" him instantly as it had the unfortunate cancer patient of years ago? Somehow, Dannie knew all along he was dying. His refusal during our sessions to bring to mind the possibility of death had indicated to me his choice, and I abided by it. But was it best for him? Was it my unconscious need rather than Dannie's that dictated my actions?

Over the next few weeks I came to see him at home two or three times weekly. During that period his weight loss and jaundice increased relentlessly, rendering a yellowed, cadaverous profile to Dannie's once full-jawed face. How much longer could he survive? Some people clung to life this way for months, lapsing into a semicomatose state, fed only intravenously and diapered and bathed like a baby. But unlike a newborn baby, no metamorphosis occurred. All that evolved was the mounting stench of feces, the pungent odor of old urine bathing an unwashed body, and the humiliation and helplessness of impending death.

Unlike many patients, Dannie remained alert, but he begged for drugs to stop his pain. Finally he became obtunded by the narcotic that diminished his physical torment and, fortunately, his sorrow. By now he was addicted to morphine and demanded it incessantly by gesture or voice. He grew less and less concerned with his family as he slept between shots, finally awakening only to plead for more drugs.

Why was death still so bitterly savage, so many centuries after the evolution of life, and why was life so obdurately unyielding? Why had nature or the nonexistent God failed to evolve a more graceful form for the inevitable? And if nature or the nonexistent God had failed, why had humankind also failed to find a way to be more merciful to itself?

Each time I saw Dannie, my anger renewed and grew to shield me and protect me, defending me against helplessness, and sorrow, and immobility.

One morning, just before I was to admit my first office patient, my phone rang. It was Florence.

"Dr. Sherwood, can you come over right away? It's Dannie. I need you."

"Is he gone, Flo?"

She gave no reply but said in a quietly urgent voice, "Please come."

"I'll be there, Flo." I wondered why she refused to tell me on the phone. Was he dead? Or was he dying at this moment? I canceled the pleasant, understanding middle-aged woman in my waiting room, expressing my regret at her inconvenience.

For one patient, today's struggle was over a minor quarrel with her son and a few harsh words from her husband, for another it was over survival itself.

Flo's face was sleeplessly haggard, wiry ringlets of hair hanging over it or sticking out from the sides of her head. "Come into the girls' bedroom. I sent the kids to my parents last night. I told them to take a last look at their daddy, but none of them wanted to go in. They've lived through enough already." Then she faced me squarely, "Dannie's dead." She waited, then went on slowly, mechanically. "He's been in constant pain, worse than when you saw him the day before yesterday. It's been one shot after another. During the day the nurse usually gives it to him but I've still been giving it to him at night. Last night he cried for pain-killers most of the night. I gave him a shot at 10 o'clock, hardly an hour after the first, and by midnight he was asking for more. Both you and Dr. Johnson said I could double the dose once in a while, so I did."

She spoke more rapidly now. "Dr. Johnson warned me to be careful, that too much could slow down his breathing so that it would be dangerous. When I saw him lying there in pain just crying for more, I put two more tablets in the syringe, but instead of giving him just those two, I put two more in, then two more, and four more, and another four, till there were no more left." Her voice cracked. "There were fifteen, maybe even twenty, in the syringe and I filled it with sterile water the way I'm supposed to." She began to sob a dry, gasping sob without tears. "And I gave him all of them, the whole syringeful, at once and I watched him lying there for a minute, and then I shut the door and left. I ran out and just drove the car around all night long." She rubbed her face. "And I didn't come back till this morning just before the nurse came on duty at seven. I opened the door and I could see he was just lying there, the way I left him. He wasn't breathing any longer—no more pain, and no more crying."

She sat down and looked up at me silently, a question in her thoughts. What would I tell the coroner when Dr. Johnson and I made out the death certificate as the physicians who had been treating Dannie? That's what occurred to me at that moment, too, and that I was glad she had done it, and that I had unconsciously wished that she would.

Autopsy was unrequired by law in the instance of a patient cared for by a physician just before death when its cause was known, and even if an autopsy were required, morphine intoxication would be difficult to detect in a patient dying of cancer and given large palliative doses of that drug.

She read my thoughts and my momentary hesitation.

"He died of his cancer, Flo. Poor Dannie. His torment is over now."

I stood there for a moment. Dannie had a secret which he withheld from Flo, and even though she suspected, she was uncertain whether or not he had broken his promise, and Flo had a secret which she withheld from Dannie. Now I had a secret, too—a secret I would withhold from society.

Sometimes when I'm awakened in the dark, cold night by the wind rustling in the birches, or by the distant, frosty barking of a dog, I find myself thinking of Dannie sleeping in the earth in silence, still hoping Flo loves him

Chapter 7
Teddy
the Fag

Teddy continued talking. We were midway through his first session. "I've never known a woman who wasn't a cunt! Oh, maybe there are a few who aren't," he said, "but most of them are such wretched creatures!"

He puffed on a cigarette as he spoke, sitting up, facing me.

"Nevertheless, they're why I'm here." He laughed slightly. "I've really got to know how to like them—the cunts! I can't go on living this way!" He waved his cigarette toward the floor in a lingering gesture of despair. "This is no life."

"So you're attracted only to men, and you seem to think about them a lot?"

"Seem." He laughed again. "Dr. Sherwood, they're all I ever think about."

"How far back in your attraction for males does your memory go?"

"To the time I was in the crib, I think—thirty-two years ago." His face lit up with a merry, yet self-abnegating, smile, as if to announce that he was good-humored even though he knew he was hopeless.

He was small with a slight build and a pleasant but plain face. His nose was straight and a bit too short, adding to his childlike appearance. His eyes were watery blue, his thin brown hair growing sparse and carefully combed over his forehead in an attempt to conceal a large bald area. He bore a clean, spice-powdered scent and an air of delicate posture whenever he moved his arms or head. Yet there was only an occasional hint of effeminacy in his mannerisms. He wore a stylish white knit sweater-shirt with wide purple stripes and a large, purple-striped kerchief around his neck which made his small head seem smaller yet.

"How far back in my attraction for males does my memory go?" he repeated, reconsidering, another mirthful, accommodating giggle coming from him. "Do I have to remember?"

As he raised his voice to express strong feelings, it assumed a peculiar, lilting intonation.

"Lord, I'm sure it was there when I was seven or eight. When I was about that old, there was an uncle I liked. He really wasn't an uncle, but my mother told me to call him that. He was simply an old family friend. One day when he visited my family, we were left alone in our house, just the two of us. I don't remember why. Maybe he was babysitting me, or maybe the rest of the family just went outside for a while. He used to come over a lot, probably to talk business with my father. I was wearing shorts, and he put his hands up my pants and began to play with me. At first I was alarmed. Then I realized I was enjoying it. Then he pulled out his dick. It was a whopper." He giggled. "It was hard and huge, and it frightened me and excited me, both. He wanted me to do something to him, but I couldn't figure out quite what. I do know I was confused and scared and titillated, and that there was something wrong with what he was doing. Now, I've finally caught on, after all these years." He laughed again.

"We lived in a little town outside of Mobile. We owned quite a few acres, and we had some people working for us, sharecroppers really. 'Niggers,' my father called them. My father had such contempt for black folks, but one of the few people I ever really loved was our Negro housekeeper. At least I think I loved her." He smiled. "She took care of me and fed me and sent me off to school. Do you suppose that's why I like only dark-complexioned men?" A titter came from him again.

I felt myself smiling. He had a sense of humor. That was a good sign, even though I suspected a depression deep within him.

"I felt so uneasy and so ashamed, and yet, a few months later I went back for more. 'Uncle Calihan'—that's what his name was—said not to tell anyone, and I didn't. I went over to his farmhouse a few times, I believe. Yes, it comes back to me now. I went back two or three times, whenever I could get my mother to send me there on an errand. He lived only a few miles away. I remember he had a big tobacco crop because I was always looking back at the huge brown-yellow leaves as

I skipped down the paths, scared someone in my family might be following me and catch us. We had cotton, corn, and a few other things growing, too.

"He wanted me to come over all the time, but I was too scared. Yet I let him play with me once in a while, and I must have enjoyed it, because I kept going back. 'Make the white stuff come out,' he'd whisper. 'Milk me, son, milk me like a cow.' And I would. Then he'd give me a quarter.

"One day, maybe I was nine or ten, I heard that he had moved away alone suddenly, leaving his wife and kids to run the farm. It wasn't till I was older, maybe twelve or thirteen, that I learned what had really happened. A couple of men caught him playing with their sons. He wasn't very faithful to me." He laughed. "They beat up on him and tarred and feathered him and rode him out of the county. Seems it wasn't the first time he'd been caught either.

"A few weeks later Uncle Calihan came back home, but people spat on him. He went to the depot and killed himself by jumping in front of the old Southern-Freight train that came through every night from Nashville. His wife, my 'aunt,' was one of my mother's best friends. I heard her whispering about it to my mother one night. Reminiscing they were, I guess. That's how I found out.

"I felt so terrible when I heard about 'Uncle Calihan' because by then I realized I was just like him and maybe partly responsible for what had happened to him. Men were terribly attractive to me, and I couldn't get what happened to him out of my mind. My Lord. I'm thirty-two now, and it seems like yesterday. For years I used to wonder if the same men who beat up my 'uncle' would find out that the Tanen boy and I were 'playing' with each other all the time. Would they rough us up and tell my parents and ride me out of town, too?

"I couldn't get the whole mess out of my mind. Night after night I couldn't sleep. I'd have nightmares, but I couldn't talk to anyone. And meanwhile, the Tanen boy and I kept jerking and sucking each other off, day after day. We couldn't stop. We'd meet in our cowshed for years. 'Such nice boys,' his mother would say. 'Real gentlemen. Never fight like all the other boys.'" Teddy laughed. "I wanted to stop. How I wanted to stop, but I couldn't—couldn't do anything about it. I just kept going back for more."

"You found it impossible to tell your father or mother?"

"My mother and father! Lord have mercy on me, no! No, no one, not even the Negro mammy whom I loved. She was the only one I could talk to, and I wouldn't dare tell her. And Mother, she was always full of pills the doctor kept giving her, long red pills and round yellow pills for sleep. Barbiturates, that's what the hospital doctors called them. She'd overdose and have to have her stomach pumped. She had all kinds of bottles full of pills lining the medicine cabinet, and she was always taking them, month after month. Sometimes she'd drink on top of it.

"And my father was usually out of it, too, by three o'clock each afternoon, dead drunk without taking any pills, and my step-sister, she was much older, and she was usually out whoring around the town and getting into her own kind of trouble—pregnant once or twice, and what not—and when she was at home she'd be constantly screaming mad at everyone. I couldn't talk to her about anything. She was never interested in me or anyone in our family. She wasn't ever home much to begin with. No, there was no one to talk to.

"Lord, I can see a typical scene—my mother sprawled on the veranda, drinking 'sasparilla' on top of her drugs, and my father staggering home from some saloon in town. He never had to work much. Some hired man ran the farm for him.

"I remember when I was little my mother would hold me on her knee and sing to me, loaded full of drugs, I suppose. My dad would be angry at her, and he'd say, 'You'll spoil that boy with all that lovin'.' I can remember for sure when I was only five because I had a party and the birthday cake had five candles in it—one for each finger of one hand, my mother pointed out. She kept begging me not to get any older, hugging and kissing me through the whole day. My dad was always cussing her out for babying me too much, but she told him to 'pay no never mind.' He was too drunk to do anything about it anyway, and she went on holding me and cuddling me like forever. I can't remember much else, except that I loved my birthdays because I always got to eat as much cake as I wanted till I got sick to my stomach and vomited.

He paused. His smile was gone. "All I want to know is, is there a chance I might like women? I feel so terribly guilty, I could vomit now, too. I just can't take it! I pick up a man in a men's bar. We drink till we're stoned, and then go to bed, and the next day it's 'ech' time. I call myself rot, and I wish I'd died in my sleep.

"And I can't go to a priest either. I want to, but I can't. How do you tell a priest and have him understand?" He clenched his fist to his forehead. His small face took on a sickly look. "How do you tell a priest you really love to suck and be sucked? And when I wake up from all that booze, with the bright sunlight shining on the ceiling of my bedroom, and I see some strange man's grimy body sleeping beside me, and I stink from sweat and alcohol, and he stinks too— and what we've done with each other all night long—it's 'ech' time! Oh, Lord in heaven, what a mess!" He looked up imploringly. The anxious, lilting quality was in his voice now.

"I used to be able to go to the priest and confess, thinking some day I would stop. Now I know I never will, and I feel rotten when I go. I even lie when I find a new priest who doesn't know me, and he asks me if it's happened before. But by now, I've used up all the priests this side of town; when they recognize me, some of them are downright mean. I can't even look to the Catholic Church anymore, the way I did when I was a kid. I've just got no one to turn to any longer." His voice broke off abruptly. His lips trembled, but no tears came. His dry eyes became lusterless and set in an unseeing gaze. A pinched, hopeless look fell over his face, which was now motionless.

I felt pressed to reassure him, but I had no basis to do so; it would have been misleading.

I broke the silence.

"Your work? You said you're a director and writer?"

"Yeah, a director who's never directed a play and a writer who's never been published—except in school. But I've almost got something now, I think. I have some pull through Irene Smith, who's talked to some producers and actors, et cetera, about my writing. What a cunt she is! Everyone in the movie industry thinks she's great, but I know the real woman behind the actress. Still, she's helping me get a job, unless I starve to death first. I'm almost broke. The only money I have is what my mother keeps sending me from the family's old, decadent farm—three or four hundred dollars a month when cotton is good—to keep me."

He shifted in his chair, the spice scent of his body floating across the room. His frozen face melted, like thin snow in a hot sun, as quickly as it had become icy. He looked up with his mild, easy smile again, revealing how adroit he was at disguising his feelings even from himself. "I'll bet you're wondering where my dialect is, for a guy who was born on a farm in the middle of Alabama."

"Yes, I did notice that you had none."

"Well, I got rid of it." He laughed. "In acting school. When I was learning to direct and write plays. All directors and writers should do some acting, too, you know. Teaches them what torment they put people through. I worked on my drawl till it was all gone, till I got all of the old South right out of me, every bit of it."

His face grew taut again.

"Do you think you can help me?"

Once more his damned demand. A guy as troubled as he was—how did I know how much he could really be helped? He was self-destructive, lonely, chronically guilt-laden, and an alcoholic—a terrible mess of a human being. He would be tough to treat, and who the hell needs another tough one? Even aside from his homosexual conflict, he desperately needed help. Maybe he could improve if he could see himself from a viewpoint other than his self-condemning morality. At least he was amusing, even likeable, this *fagella*, this tender fag.

"In all probability, you'll feel better with treatment, but how much your sexual feelings can change is a question only time can answer. I'm willing to see you five days a week, if we can arrange to meet that often. The real problem will be to see why your life has become what it has, and how much damned hard work you are willing to do to change it.

No magic solution. I let him know right from the start. There had been omnipotent moments in my career when I believed that I might chance upon some unusual creation, some heretofore undiscovered meandering of the mind that no one had dreamed of before this hour. But the years had dashed this hope.

I almost wished, as I had before with patients as difficult as Teddy, that I had remained in general medicine, where there was a formulated treatment for a given disease and the responsibility for success or failure after a clever diagnosis rested not with me, but with a life-maintaining agent like cortisone, or a hormone combination needed to cure a deficiency disease, or a life-saving antibiotic, an indifferent-looking colored powder queezed into a capsule. To hell with all this pressure.

Have no therapeutic ambition, I was taught. Nonsense. Why treat a patient if there is no hope for improvement? But who needed this much tension?

The patient looked up a little startled and then smiled again. "So you're going to make me work, eh? I've heard about that old game. Well, I've got to do something, and I might as well do this. Doctor, do you really think there's a chance I might have a woman?"

"That depends on many things, Teddy, including how really strong your wish to change is."

"The only time it's strong, Doctor, is at 'ech' time." He laughed. He took his appointment card. "Then Wednesday we'll discuss when we're going to meet and what you charge and all that, you said? OK. See you then. Lord, I hope this works."

"I have a grant from the university to do some part-time research in the area of homosexuality," I explained. "Your fee will be twenty dollars per meeting. The research grant will pay me the rest. It's part of a large study with a number of psychiatrists participating."

"How much will they pay you?"

"Enough to bring the fee to nearly average for patients in this area. I enjoy doing research, so the fee is enough to satisfy me."

He seemed relieved. Now we could begin individual work.

"What kind of study? What do I have to do?"

"Your job and mine will be to try to discover something more of the etiology of the problem of homosexuality by a long-term, in-depth study. We'll work in therapy in a confidential relationship as I would with any other patient. The research will be a by-product of the pooled observations gathered by the doctors involved."

"Good." He was grinning. "I've always wanted to be a subject in a scientific study. At least I'll be of some use to humanity, because if this doesn't work, I've made up my mind to kill myself, and you can use my case to learn more about why people like me kill themselves. So you want me just to go on and say whatever comes to mind about myself? I don't know where to begin."

"Tell me more about your life at the present time," I said.

After several weeks: "Today and yesterday and all my days are usually the same," he began one day. "I go to the studios looking for work. I told you I'm trying to finish a play, a comedy. I'm good at writing comedies, but I haven't done much work this last year or so, I feel so lousy all the time.

"Irene's still trying to sell it to one of the producers who did her last movie. She's really been pushing for me. She wants to play the lead in it. I wrote the script a long time ago. It won first place in a national college contest, and it was published in a collection of university students' plays, but it was never put on anywhere. I've rewritten a lot of it to improve it in places, and the stupid studio's interested in it. That's the main thing.

"It's about a selfish nephew who comes back home to a little farming town trying to get his uncle's will changed so he can get more of his money when he dies. He even tries to wheedle a loan from his uncle or steal from him. Finally, he's joined in a plot with another cousin, a woman—that's Irene—to kill the senile old man, but then everything gets loused up, and it turns into a big farce because the uncle himself unwittingly joins the plot without realizing he's the one they're out to get. It's not quite a classic Italian comedy, but it could turn out good if they'll only let me redo it the way I want to.

"Oh well, the studios may pay something just to get an option on the manuscript. People say I'm clever and sensitive and original and all that rot." His cheeks pinched and he took on a pained look momentarily. "But it's tough for any new writer to get a real chance, ever. The closest I've come, besides winning that college prize, was when one of my later plays almost sold to a Broadway producer before he got scared and backed out. He was afraid a new writer couldn't draw an audience, even though he loved my script."

His pleasant smile slowly returned. "In the last few years I nearly sold a few TV scripts for stupid comedy shows. 'Nearly sold' and 'almost a success' is my middle name." He laughed. "But I hate that kind of work. Writing for TV is the lowest form of human existence. It's so degrading," he said with exaggerated horror, "but not having money to pay my rent," he laughed again, "is even more degrading. So I became a TV script prostitute instead of a male homosexual prostitute, as if I've had any offers lately."

He smiled brightly now. "So here I am, running back and forth to New York. What I really want to do is to write and direct my own plays and movies, but there's not much chance of that. All they want is stupid, light comedy junk. Still, Irene's a big name in movies, you know, and whatever she touches turns into diamonds and platinum, not just gold, except when she touches me. I turn into instant hate." His eternal little laugh arose again. "She uses me as if I were her valet and her servant extraordinaire.

"How did I get to know her? She's from the South, too. Her mother and mine were childhood girl friends. Her mother lives in town here. My mother asked her mother to introduce us ten years ago. Since then, Irene and I have been close in a way. Every time she gets divorced she comes crying to me, and I escort her to parties and gatherings so she won't be alone, and I let her cry on my shoulder like a best girl friend would. She's been married four times—no, five, counting the annulment of her last marriage to that oil magnate, Timothy Willington Donahue. She never really dug him—only his oil.

"She treats me like a woman, walks around nude in front of me when she's bathing and dressing, and even asks me to give her a rubdown. Ech!" he laughed. "—cover her all over with banana and avocado oil and rub her down! And then I smell for a week like bananas and avocados. But I'd jump into a barrel of cow manure and rub her down with it if she asked me to—that's how low and desperate I am. She even asks me to fix her hair, or at least go with her to the beauty shop so I can make sure they do it right.

"People are beginning to call her a second Marilyn Monroe— another blonde bombshell. Well, I can vouch that she is a natural blonde—the only natural or real thing about her.

"She says I'm the only friend she can trust—the cunt. Women always stab her in the back, she says. And men find her either very sexy or intolerable, and, after she marries them, mostly intolerable. She's got a quick and vicious temper, like my sister, and she's got to have her own way in everything, never ever listens to anyone else's opinion about anything, and just uses people. I don't know how I stand her. She's really the one in my play I'd like to kill, not the poor old uncle, but if I kill her off, she'll have no part and I'll have no chance to sell my play." He smiled. "And no 'good' friend to bathe and rub down. Lord, I'm beginning to hate myself for using people the way she does, but I am becoming proficient at it."

"So," I said, "she's tough to deal with, but you have to take her, huh?"

"I'll say. I'd take anything from her. I'm so hungry and down-and-out, I'd kneel in back of her with my hands cupped and make like a toilet if she wanted me to. Still, if I were the uncle in the play, I'd try to kill her instead of the other way around. In fact, I think I'll change it to that at the end of the script. Maybe I'm beginning to understand this crazy movie I've written after all." He giggled.

"Oh well, at least she doesn't condemn me for my feelings about men. She knows all about me, and at the moment, I think we're both falling in love with the same man, the director of her last picture, Anthony de Mitrelli. She thinks he's great. What she doesn't know yet is that he's one of us, just like lots of other directors and actors and producers. Usually, everyone in the theatrical business knows who's gay and who's straight, but he's managed somehow to keep it a secret—maybe because he's divorced. He got married to throw everyone off the track, but I know because another actor friend of mine—a young kid of twenty-three—and he have been living together. De Mitrelli's forty-seven—a beautiful man with dark eyes and olive-colored skin, just greying a little. But he's not mine, so who cares anyway?"

His face grew unsmiling, revealing the depression that his smiles tried to hide.

I felt his real despair at this moment. I noticed that I avoided looking directly into his eyes. I dreaded seeing the disappointment that would someday appear in them and spread across his shocked face, for now I was nearly certain a woman would never arouse him erotically. It was rare, if ever, for a man whose sensual feelings for males were of such long duration and intensity as Teddy's to develop a heterosexual lust.

There was an aura of solitude—a sadness surrounding the small being of this gentle man. And in these feelings were hidden the genesis of his alcoholism, his isolation, his lack of self-regard, and his deep anger, the anger that raged only when he was drunk.

I loved obstetrics. Helping to bring infants down an intriguing canal was an erotic pleasure in itself. And afterward the squirming baby filled me with the excitement and hope of a new life moving in my hands, and a mother grateful for the relief of her pain and the gift of a child. As if I had really done something. It was so simple.

For a few moments after birth, the infant screeches with clutched fists and curled toes, flapping and flailing its limbs angrily, but with sensible attention paid to its natural wants, it becomes content and is soon asleep in its mother's lap, a sweet, uncomplicated psyche beginning a career never lived before and never again to be repeated by anyone. (Yet this was how some of them end up.)

Delivering a baby was a joy. Delivering an adult like Teddy from his neurotic hell was devilish. So let him stay in hell. But then, I argue with myself, what could be more intriguing than the eternally changing enigmas inside the skull of a complex patient with a history of having endured? Bullshit, Sherwood!

I laughed at myself when I called him "fag." It was a remnant of my childhood fear and disdain for homosexuals—a contempt for them, a convenient vehicle to disguise from myself my doubts and fears about my own masculinity.

When I was thirteen, I was careful to walk with a male swagger. I had heard that fairies had a girlish gait, and even in recent years with all my enlightenment, I wondered if my medical colleagues would think I had a gross mental aberration, even being queer, which drew me into psychiatry. After my decision to switch into this field, I went out of my way to chat with some of them to demonstrate my "normalcy."

Sergeant Schultz had to ridicule and humiliate men to show how fearsomely manly he was. When we caught an SS paratrooper captain alone in the woods after a battle, Schultz slapped him in the face and told him we were going to shoot him on the spot. This was the fierce, masculine sadism that wars allow, even foster and praise, as good soldiering.

There were only three of us there in a grove of the dense Black Forest of Germany—Schultz, Wollman, and I. With a challenging snarl, Schultz threw the SS captain a short rope that he had used to tie some K-rations together and said he could hang himself if he wanted to. "We hang SS men anyway," Schultz informed him with a grim smile.

The SS man broke away and ran wildly, trying to lose us in the woods. Schultz calmly opened up with his grease gun and pumped a full magazine of cartridges after the fleeing man. His chopped body lay only twenty steps away from us when we found him.

Schultz then turned to the two of us and said, "You guys saw him run, didn't you?" And we reported: the prisoner tried to run. My anger at the cruel SS permitted me to do it—let me justify Schultz's murder, Schultz's unconscionable brutality.

Anger arose to color Teddy's sadness with a tinge of orange flush when he began again. "I've lived with several different men in my lifetime—the last one, Larry, for about a year, the longest ever. I thought I loved him deeply," Teddy said, meditatively, "and I even thought he loved me. Larry was four years younger than I. I met him from hanging out around the theater. He was an actor.

"One day when my back was turned, he left me for another actor he'd met—a kid of twenty-two, fresh and new to the game. You see, there are very few lasting relationships among us homosexuals. But then," he said, smiling, "there aren't very many among heterosexuals either. So I go back again and again to the bars and to the homosexual parties and hangouts or to the baths and try to pick someone up, someone attractive or at least halfway appealing to me.

And older men try to pick me up—men in their fifties and even sixties—while I'm trying to pick up some young kid in his twenties. It's all a very sad, sad scene when you get up in years, unless you're famous and good-looking like de Mitrelli, until he gets a few years older, too, and nobody wants him either, except some gigolo. This town's loaded with gigolos looking to be supported by rich old geezers."

He paused. "There's no fag like an old fag." Then he looked up with a half-humorous, half-somber face. "Larry and I had lots in common. He loved the theater and good movies, and he had a degree in theater arts from Alabama, same as I do. He acted in university plays and summer stock. He really never was very good, except at comedies, the times I saw him. We had plans once for me to write and direct one just for him to be the lead, hoping we could get it put on somewhere, some day. Comedy is what we both liked best. I can't be serious for too long, you know. It hurts too much." He grinned. "So we'd sit for hours in our apartment, night after night, and dream of how we would make it big together. And for a while we were a happy couple. But whenever we got to drinking, I'd grow morose and start crying.

"Sometimes when I was drunk, I'd feel so bad I wanted to do away with myself for no reason that I could understand. Maybe it was because I began to see the truth when I drank. Down deep I knew that none of our dreams would ever come true. And he was too good-looking. I knew someone would steal him away from me sooner or later, and I'd be alone again. I fall in love only with good-looking men, and they're the first to be stolen away, or the first to leave you for somebody else."

He waited for a moment and said, "A gay man is the loneliest guy on heaven and earth." I caught a glimpse of the concealed anger that transformed his face into a momentary taut mask.

"You place a lot of importance on good looks and youth," I said without thinking. Was I being conciliatory? I regretted saying it.

"Who doesn't in our world, yours or mine?" he shot back. "It hurts to even think about him." He set his teeth and waved his smoking cigarette downward in his gloomy gesture. "The man I loved was nearly six feet tall, with a theatrical jutting jaw and deep blue eyes and a trim yet muscular build like a football player—not a lineman, but a quarterback. I don't know anything about football. Quarterbacks are the ones that aren't too big, someone once told me. The roughest game I ever played was ping-pong." Out came his easy-flowing laugh again.

"Anyway, I suspected—no, I knew all along—he was just a small-time, amateur gigolo. The only reason he lived with me is because I paid the rent and all the upkeep. Everything he ever said to me was just a lie." He waved his cigarette toward the floor once more, a look of futility settling again on his face. "I keep thinking, though, that I must really have been in love with him. I still can't get him out of my mind.

"Funny thing." His face lit up. "I just remembered this. Whenever we got drunk, I would sit him on my knee and talk baby talk to him . . ."

"Baby talk?"

"Yeah. Seems to me now I even sounded like my mother when she would sit me on her lap. Lord! I think I even used some of the same words she would use—'My little teddy bear, my sweet, sweet, little bunny-bear-boy,' and she'd rock me and hold me close and cuddle and love me. Why, I haven't thought about what she said to me in years—I just did it with Larry—I never even thought about it. I'd be drunk, and I never realized till now—I'd play mother to him."

"You were unconsciously reenacting her. You say she'd sit for hours that way with you?"

"Yeah. Even when I was nearly eight or nine or maybe even ten. I was practically an only child. My sister was eight years older, from my dad's first marriage. His first wife drowned in the Gulf of Mexico. She was on a pleasure cruise for a weekend, supposedly with a friend, but I heard from an aunt, when I was seventeen, that she was out with another man. My aunt even made inferences that the other man, not my dad, had fathered my sister, and that my dad knew it, but never said anything to his wife. He was afraid of accusing her. He was a timid kind of guy—timid and scared of being left to live alone. He was always cold and aloof toward my sister. The rumor was probably true, and he knew it. I had such a screwed-up family!

"Well, the whole boat sank, and my sister's mother and a bunch of people were never heard from again—so six months later he married my mother. He hoped she'd help bring up my sister, who was only two or three then, but my mother just ignored both of them, my dad said. The only thing my mother ever wanted, she told everyone, was a boy of her own, but people said she acted as if what she really wanted was a daughter or a doll, and it seems to me they were right. She called me her 'blue-eyed, sweet, lovely darling' and 'Teddy-bunny-bear-boy' and words like that even when I got older, and I never could get her to stop hugging and babying me.

"It began to sicken me! By the time I was nine or ten, I hated her for doing it. I tried to get away from her—no, not really—I guess I loved her, too. She seemed so sad if I didn't want to go to her that I felt I had to, whether I liked it or not.

"She's never moved from our old house, and she still uses a lot of barbiturates and all kinds of other sleeping stuff along with heavy drinking. She's been in and out of hospitals for drug overdose again and again from the time I was a small child, as far back as I can remember. Each time she does it, her doctor swears that the next time will be her last, but she manages, somehow, to live through it and sleep it off, and she goes back home to do it all over again a month or two later."

He continued in our next session.

"My dad—he was never around much, and when he was, he was drunk. I never really got to know him till my later childhood—a few years before he died. He developed a serious liver disease from all those years of drinking and had to stay home.

"I still remember one of the few things he ever said to me just before he passed away. I was in my teens by then. He always felt so lonely, and I guess he knew he was going soon. 'Life is a strange puzzle,' he said. 'There are always people around you and still you're all alone, and lots of things happen to you that no one can explain, from the day you're born till the day you die. I could never understand what life was all about.' And neither can I.

"I never asked him what he meant by 'strange puzzle,' but I guess now maybe he meant having a need for someone to love like his first wife and not being loved in return. Or maybe he meant he wasn't ever able to love anyone or anything except alcohol. I know he didn't love my mother. He never did. He never really loved any of us. He just married her to keep from feeling so desolate, and to have someone to take care of my sister."

He looked deliberately at me. "Do you love your wife?"

His unexpected question startled me. None of your fucking business, I thought of saying. That would bring a laugh.

I reflected for a moment on the vicissitudes of my marriage, of the times of closeness and the times when I wished that my wife and I had never met, and I daydreamed of someone else who was less grudging and more tolerant of my interests: "Work, work is all you ever do. When do you have time for your family?" she demanded when she was irritated. Her accusations stung me sharply.

Likewise, I had been disgruntled with her on dozens and dozens of occasions for a variety of reasons. Many times I had to remind myself to dismiss my infantile wounded anger or hurt, lest they fester too long and destroy our relationship. Teddy's perceptiveness had struck home. In a lucid moment like this, I could recognize that in ways I was unreasonable in my demands or too preoccupied with my own endeavors. She had cause to be resentful.

"Are there many men," his attack persisted, "who still love their wives after years of marriage?"

How many could there be, I wondered? He had reason to look with skepticism into the very warp of the tapestry in which many unions became entwined; they were a patchwork of the unresolved frustrations of childhood and the demands and irritations of married life, wherein dangling threads of charges and countercharges of past offenses were interwoven with the strife of recent times to create a tangled mosaic of half truths and half lies.

After waiting a long while, Teddy realized that I chose to remain silent. His serious and suspicious look changed to a grin.

Was it a triumphant look? Had he detected something of my thoughts, something of my embarrassment?

To hell with him again. The answer was yes. Reasonable men can love reasonable women and be loved in turn for a lifetime, if there is enough sincerity and flexibility between them, and some self-awareness; and fags can love each other, too. Older lovers may lose passion but they have a repertoire of shared memories and occasionally even a friendship. But I said nothing. I only looked back at him. He was baiting me. He had done this many times before, seeking to defeat me, seeking to defeat himself so that he could quit his struggle and sink back into the alcoholism from which he was emerging. His ultimate surrender would be to suicide.

I'll make you fight, wretched Teddy, ex-teddy-bear-boy, till you decide to spare yourself, I thought.

Like Abraham about to sacrifice Isaac when the angel of mercy stayed his hand, you must spare yourself because you deserve no hateful self-death. (Wasn't Abraham's struggle really an unconscious struggle over whether or not he was worthy, and whether or not he deserved to suffer the most terrible loss of all?)

"I guess," he finally said, "you want me to answer the question about people loving me for myself." I nodded yes.

The months passed. Teddy continued to work on himself, delving into the unconscious and conscious aspects of his character formation, attempting to understand his past and present attitude toward life. His guilty feelings over his homosexual impulses were probed again and again as he attempted to trace his sinful affects to their origins.

Teddy glared at me unexpectedly in the middle of a session. "I hate you," he said. "Sometimes for a second or two I feel that I just hate you." His upper lip was drawn back, exposing his teeth in the manner of a snarling cat. His face lost its boyish look for a moment. "It's when you begin to remind me how I felt when my mother wanted too much of me, especially when you seem too interested, even though you want me to get well. Don't ask me how," he said, relaxing and smiling, "you can seem too interested. I thought those feelings wouldn't happen because I expected them, but they happen anyway. And then I realize that you aren't my mother, or the priest, or anyone else, just you. And then I'm always expecting you to damn me or preach to me, too. Sometimes I think I wouldn't care so much any more even if you did. . . ."

During many other sessions he returned to his attacks on me. He was working out some feelings in terms of me.

One day there began a small but important variation in his associations. "I keep wondering about marriage," he said. "Any kind of marriage between any two people. I mean, can someone really be happy with another person? I've always wanted to be happy with a woman if I could be, but now I'm thinking, if I have a right to, even with a man. Am I beginning to feel that way lately, or am I just thinking it?

"All this thinking and talking about my life is beginning to drive me crazy. Poor old Uncle Calihan keeps coming back to my mind now. I can't get rid of him. He had a strange urge to play with little boys, but did he deserve to die? He worked hard all his life and never did anything else wrong. That's what puzzled everyone.

"And I've never even harmed one soul—but myself. I tell you, my thoughts are making me dizzy. I can't get things straight in my mind any more—what's right and what isn't. It's driving me insane." His sparse eyebrows arched high over his blue eyes as his small face reddened and screwed itself up to one side, giving him a comical appearance though he was as serious as I had ever seen him.

"Why shouldn't I be entitled to love a man if that's the way I feel? Why should I have to drink to forget myself? I feel better on the days when I don't begin all that drinking. In my later years, I've often begun feeling terrible about myself till I have some booze, but with it I feel even more wretched. Can I really stop? ..."

A month later, we scheduled a two-week break from our work so that Teddy could be at a movie studio for daily meetings, which his agent had finally arranged with Irene's producers.

A severe jury of studio heads had become interested in some of his work and were debating its acceptance.

Teddy knew that most scripts which swamped the offices of studios, even those that evoked enthusiasm, were ultimately rejected.

Then came our first meeting following the break.

"They signed me on!" he blurted as he darted in, waving a sheath of rolled papers above his head. He continued yelling, "They finally signed a contract to buy my movie script—the one about the scurrilous nephew, that crazy comedy. I've finally got a contract and a check, twenty-four thousand dollars cash for the script and twenty-four thousand more when the final version is done, plus two percent of the gross—a marvelous beginning, and I think it was my writing, not just Irene, even though she's starring in it. Sure, her pull helped me get them to read it, but they loved my writing." His voice lowered unexpectedly. "Oh yes, there was also a disaster along with all the marvelous things that took place since I last saw you—one horrid calamity."

He puckered his thin, trembling lips. Then he bit the inside of his cheek, a mannerism I had not seen before in him. The lilt in his voice, under this extreme tension, was decidedly girlish.

"It was terrible—an absolute disaster!"

He saw the puzzlement in my face. Before I could say anything, he continued, shouting. "We were celebrating my contract." He danced a few steps in a small circle. "The studio signed me on—a miracle! They're even thinking of me being assistant director, at no extra pay, just to get the experience, and Irene said I should celebrate. This was the time. On a foolish, utterly foolish whim of the moment, I agreed, and Irene fixed me up. I would have agreed to float into the sky on a soap bubble or to marry the ugly, selfish nephew in my movie if she told me to."

After a moment: "I should have known better. But I was willing to try anything, I was so happy! So she fixed me up," he caught his breath, "with a starlet girl friend of hers, a newcomer, to try sex with. She thought this would be the right time—in a moment of triumph. I've really got a contract," he repeated, reaching into his pocket to pull out the papers he had already tucked away, flipping them in the air again. "Well, we tried it, and it was a disaster. It was more than a disaster—it was a tragedy with some of the trappings of a comedy, except that I was 'it'—King Lear and Hamlet, Falstaff and Polonius, all rolled into one humiliated bundle of flaccid flesh, and flaccid I remained.

"She was good-looking enough and nice enough—at first. 'Get it on,' she kept saying, 'get it on,' and she took my little member—where in the world did she ever get that name?—and kept tugging at it and jerking at it, once so violently I thought it would rip right off.

"It was Irene's idea for me to try sex with a woman, a stranger who wouldn't threaten me, to see if I could, at last. Well, she didn't threaten me. She almost killed me! I couldn't do it with a friend or someone I knew, I told Irene. So she reached for the phone and in half an hour got this starlet she knew—not a prostitute—no, not for money, just a girl trying to do Irene a favor, and, I guess, trying to help her own career in the movies.

"When the starlet arrived at Irene's house, Irene left. The girl got undressed, and there I was—all alone with a naked twenty-four-year-old model. I felt nothing, as usual. Looking at her bare breasts and her privates stimulated me about as much as a nude statue made of marble would. She even spread the lips of her pussy to try to arouse me, but that red slimy area didn't interest me in the slightest. I wasn't horrified at it the way some gay guys are—just uninterested. And then she tried to stuff me in, but nothing, absolutely nothing, happened. I just lay there all shriveled up and couldn't stand her touching me.

"If I were simply watching that scene in a movie, I would have thought it was one of the funniest I'd ever seen, but it was happening to me, and I could hardly laugh, it was so tragic, and at the same time so comical.

"And then she got irritated at me and started carping at me and my little member. That was hardly calculated to make my little member cooperative, and it made me feel angry. What the hell was it to her? Then I refused to let her even come near me. I was ready to scream for Irene." He laughed. "I knew that by now she was undoubtedly plotting to grab me and hold me down while she attempted to rape me. It was frightening. Oh, it wasn't the first time I've ever tried it with a woman—once when I was a kid of seventeen or eighteen, and I couldn't do anything then either, but we thought, really Irene thought, that with nearly a year of therapy, I should try it again.

"It sounded crazy to me," his tone fell, "but I let her go ahead anyway while I didn't have a chance to think it over or back out, hoping she could catch me by surprise with my pants down, so to speak. Such a stupid idea. Just because I've finally sold a script." A quick smile when he touched his script alternated with a tense, puckered-lip, momentary anguish. Then came a look of confusion, suddenly replaced by a brightened look of excited triumph, then by one of anguish again.

Now he looked up at me fully, his smooth face greying and filled with doubt. "I'm never going to be able to make love to women, Dr. Sherwood! You know it and I know it, so why pretend? A year ago I'd have felt like killing myself right now because I know there's no hope of that. But I feel I'm beginning to hate myself a little less.

"Once, a long time ago, I even bought a revolver and loaded it and put it inside my mouth. I never told you this before. I didn't want to frighten you." He smiled. "But I figured if therapy didn't work ...

"I was afraid to pull the trigger then, and I've decided now I'm not going to, ever. And furthermore," he chuckled momentarily, "the noise would frighten me too much, and our research project would be doomed. And most important," he said, smiling slightly. "I've become too valuable to the world of science to be killed."

He was silent for a moment. "I know I won't ever be able to love a woman—or even make love to one. But I'm not responsible for what I feel about men and women, and besides, I probably never should have condemned myself in the first place. The Catholic Church be damned."

He paused again in thoughtful silence. "At least I don't hate myself so much." He lit a cigarette, puffing on it once or twice. Then he held it between his fingers motionlessly. "What a crazy thing to do. Lord." He laughed. "It was such an embarrassing thing to do, and she tried so hard to arouse me, this girl, and we kept trying, and trying, as I said, ..."

And our work continued.

Chapter 8
Obsessive Boy

The child sat in my consulting room kicking his feet, moving his legs, and tossing his head from side to side. He appeared to be seven or eight years old. His parents said he was eleven. He was gaunt with a thin face and dark, tense eyes that bulged out of his restless, swaying head. Both parents waited gloomily.

"Can't you ever stop?" his mother asked as she pointed to his fidgeting. She addressed her remarks to no one in particular. "He never seems to be able to stop, even here." The father paid no attention to her. He sat staring into space.

The boy stood up, pointed to the curtains, and said, 'What's behind there?' He moved the curtains back and peered behind them. Then he went to the window and looked out, saying, "Our car is over there." Then he sat down again, tapped the floor with his fingers, arose again, sat down, tapped the floor again, and resumed his former posture, fidgeting. Mother looked at him with a pained expression. Father continued looking into nowhere.

"My God," said Mother, "what are we going to do with him?"

Father sat still, despondent and silent again as if she had said nothing. Finally he spoke, "How did he ever get that way? How did he ever get that way?"

The boy's pallor was apparent despite his dark-complexioned skin. He listened as his parents gave their history.

"He's always asking questions," Mother said. "In fact, people call him 'Mr. Questions.'"

As if responding to Mother's cue, the child looked at me and said, "How old are you? Are you married? Do you have any children? What time is it?"

"See?" his mother said. "He's always asking questions, even when they don't make sense—as if out of a clear blue sky. He can be watching television, and then he'll look up and say something that just doesn't make sense."

The father interjected with a touch of pride to compensate for his pain, "But he always knows what's going on, and he can always tell you about the television program. In fact, he has an unusually good memory."

They both looked at the boy, who shook his head and said, "I can't remember much," and again began to fire a barrage of questions.

The mother said, "He can remember telephone numbers, dates, birthdays, all kinds of things."

The boy interrupted, looking at me, "Do you know any birthdays in August?"

"He's a real worrier," his mother said. "Even when he was small, he would shake and tremble if any stranger came near him, and he would wake up at night and cry all the time. He was scared of nightmares, and strange noises, and shadows in the dark, and what could happen to him. I think he still worries about some of those things, even now. Don't you, honey?" she said in a sympathetic tone, knowing full well his many fears.

The child ignored her words. He rubbed his hands together and touched my desk, then folded his hands in his lap for a moment.

"You must have wondered about what all his worries mean?" I asked.

"Well, maybe we worry a little too much ourselves," she said, looking at Father.

"I guess that's right. I do worry—but," Father emphasized, "just about normal things. Like when I drive to work every day to the plant and I see all that speeding crazy traffic, and all the kinds of strange people who live in a big city like Los Angeles. That's no place for a little kid to be wandering in alone. Maybe we were a little strict, but we had to watch him, specially with the kinds of things people think and do in a big city. I come from a God-fearing small farming town in Virginia. That's the place to grow up—with good Baptist people who teach their children right from wrong—lots of mischief and bad things in crowded neighborhoods. So we didn't let him wander all around like other little kids when he was growing up, getting into all kinds of trouble." He laughed feebly. "Maybe we were too careful."

"Yes, maybe we were a little strict," Mother said. "My own mother and father, they were real strict, and they never let their children talk back like kids do nowadays, and we didn't want our children to talk back to us either."

"No," Father said. "He's a real good boy. He never talks back."

"That's right," Mother agreed. "He never talks back and he minds us real good, except when he fidgets and won't stop and when he asks all those silly questions."

"But it isn't the questions that bother us so much," said the father. "It's the things that bother him—like praying at night. Now it takes him two hours to say his prayers, and every time he gets to the word 'God' he's got to repeat it four or five times, and then he asks us, 'Did I say that right? Does God believe me? Does God think I'm bad? Does God make anybody hurt?' It's so painful with his prayers that we asked him to stop altogether."

"That's right," Mother said. "We asked him to stop, but he just keeps on going with the prayers and never wants to stop."

I asked the parents to leave. Then I asked the boy about his prayers and what else worried him.

The boy rubbed his hands together several times, looked up, then again touched the floor and the corner of my desk. He touched it twice and then put his hands back in his lap, and then touched it twice more, and put his hands back in his lap again.

"That must mean something to you," I said.

He nodded his head and mumbled.

"You have lots of worries, don't you?"

"Yes, I worry sometimes. Do you know any birthdays in August? Are you married? Do you have any children?"

"Tell me more about the things you worry about, Billy."

He looked hesitant.

"I'd like to help you, you know."

He seemed to understand. "I worry about my parents."

"What sort of things?"

He looked around the room and said, "I worry about my parents." Then he looked behind the curtain and sat again in his seat.

"Are you worried about their health, that something might happen to them, Billy?"

He looked relieved and said, "Yes, I worry that they might die. I worry all the time when they're gone and even when they're home. I don't like my mother to sit too close to the window 'cause I heard of something crashing through the window once and hurting somebody.

That's why I make sure she sits away from the window. Then I go into the corner and pray, just the way my mind tells me to."

"What else does your mind tell you to do?"

"My mind tells me to go into the corner and pray so that I won't have any worries. I pray that my mother and father won't get hurt and that nobody else in the family will get hurt."

"What other kind of thoughts do you have about your parents?"

"I think good things about them. I want my mother to have good things. I think only good things."

"You mean you never let yourself think bad things about them? What if you get mad at them?"

"When they get mad at me, they yell at me and I say, 'Stop yelling.'"

"And then?"

"Then it's over."

"So you never get mad at them?"

"I think only good things about them."

"So you can't have any bad thoughts, can you?"

"No, I only think good things about them," the boy persevered.

"Even when they get mad and yell at you?"

"Well, sometimes they get mad at me," the boy faltered and then quickly added, "but I never get mad at them."

"So you can only think good things about them and if any bad thoughts come up you have to do something with your hands or say your prayers so nothing bad will happen to them."

He looked stunned for a moment and then nodded his head affirmatively, touched the floor twice, then the corner of the desk, and rubbed his hands. He looked behind the curtain again.

"What do you think is behind there?" I asked.

"I was just checking."

"You look pretty worried about it."

"Well, I was just checking. Once I read about something coming from behind a curtain and doing something to people."

"So you have to keep checking to make sure that it's all right."

The boy, displaying his good intelligence, nodded and said, "How can I stop this? I don't know how to stop. I want to stop, but I can't. I don't know how."

"Maybe I can help you to stop. Let me talk to your parents for a few moments."

The boy stepped out, and his parents came back in hesitantly.

Mother interrupted my brief explanation. "You mean he's so worried about doing bad things and thinking bad things that he prays? And all them silly questions have meanings?"

"My God, how did he ever get that way?" the father said.

"What can we do about it?" Mother said.

I indicated the kind of treatment the boy needed.

Both parents seemed to understand a little bit about it and readily agreed that the boy needed some sort of help.

"But he's always been so good," the father said. "He does everything just the way he should—not like some boys. He never says bad things and he never does bad things. We just want him to not have to pray so much or worry so much."

The boy entered again and sat down near his parents.

"Stop that shaking," the father said, looking up. Then he rubbed his own head and said, "Sorry, I can't help talking to him when he shakes like that! My God, how did he get that way?"

The child stood up, looked out the window again, and then looked apprehensively at Mother. He sat down, rubbed his hands, touched the floor, rubbed his hands again, and again touched the floor.

Both parents looked at me.

"That's all right," his father said. "I understand from what you say it means something to him, and maybe we can help him understand so someday he can stop if he wants to."

The boy looked relieved, sat back in his chair, and stared blankly into space. He seemed to rest for a few moments. Then he seemed to awaken startled, began to fidget again, looked about the room, sighed heavily, and said, "Do you know any birthdays in August? Are you married? Do you have any children?"

"Mr. Questions," Mother said.

The father, again appearing puzzled and glum, looked at me, then at Mother, and said, "My God, how did he get that way?" Then he turned his gaze away from us and stared straight ahead with weary resignation.

Chapter 9
Emma in
the Rest Home

One night I saw my mother dying. I awakened smothered by a sense of despair that enveloped me like a dense, unremitting fog.

Five years before, my mother had become ill, her kind, full face slowly growing narrow and linear, her hair scraggly-thin and white. Despite my medical knowledge, I stood by in helpless anguish.

After her illness began, she grew too weak to care for herself. I placed her in the Seaside Rest Home, the most caring and the best home in the West, they claimed. There for months she lingered in painful heart failure, gasping and struggling to live. Or was it to die? I was deeply relieved one night to find her in final sleep, her mouth half-open as in her last breath.

Since her death, I had fought to keep out of mind the sorrowful ending of her life.

Immediately following my dream, the coldness of my head and face was replaced by a heated flushing and sweating. I remembered that the next morning I was scheduled to visit a patient at the same rest home, where I had been so many times before to see my mother or to consult on other patients.

My heavy sense of sadness blanketed me for hours. I managed to brush it aside and fall asleep again.

The next morning I arrived at the Seaside.

The hallway bore the characteristic odor of the elderly, the sick, and the unwashed feeble. Although the dayrooms had ample space and light, the tubular steel chairs, the silent, swift elevators, the metallic groan of the electrically operated beds gave the place an air of detachment—the mechanical somberness of twentieth-century death.

In an isolated sector, the sterile, white-clothed disinfectant-smelling nurses bustled about, chattering in clipped, esoteric medical phrases to one another, while charting and answering telephones with the fervor of a stock-exchange operation—where phone orders are translated into actions of buying, though all that could be purchased here was the pretense of prolonging life. The week's or month's losses were tallied by the occasional beds that were rolled inconspicuously down the hallways, usually at night, sheets and blankets draped over a body, an ashen face exposed. Here and there, from a doorway, came a silent, hollow-socket stare from an elderly face, transfixed by the specter of the inevitable journey.

The shabby-trousered orderly usually employed for this task slowly pushed his charge, smiled a nodding hello to the onlookers, and said reassuringly, "It's just a change of rooms for old Mr. Alfred. He'll be able to lie more comfortably in the special room where he's going." These words, intended to avoid frightening the viewers, contained, I thought, a mocking sadism.

I felt enraged at him—or was my fury at death's insensitivity?

I tried to read the chart of my patient, to shut out the words penetrating the hallway, when I saw my mother's face drifting toward me again. My sorrow returned, this time refusing to leave, rising fully to consciousness as it swept over me in another wave of grief. How inured and indifferent I had grown to loneliness and death. They had lived so close to me during my day-in, day-out tasks that they had clearly become partners, companions to my existence, no longer the great and hated enemies I had fought during my early years of medicine. At one time I had a vigorous and incalculable belief in my ultimate victory, when I felt that intensity of purpose and knowledge could make the difference. What had become of this precious faith? Where had I mislaid it?

The nurses and patients seemed unaware of me as I sat silently, out of view, in the doctors' alcove. Now I was listening intently.

"There's a new patient named Emma in 124," the head nurse said wearily. "She's in with the thin old woman and Violet, the woman with the stroke. They won't be much company or help to a new patient, so we might as well get that new one settled for her first night here."

Emma's daughter, Terry, had brought her mother to me a few

weeks before to consult on the family doctor's evaluation. Terry held a handkerchief to her eyes, her face swollen from crying, bulging veins arabesquing down her long, thin neck. While she and I were alone, she had described in detail her life with her aging mother. Then she had confided to me that she had been vomiting continually during the last few days, sickened by her feeling that she was abandoning her mother.

Emma had told me, as the tears rolled down her cheeks, of her life with her only child. During the preceding weeks, I came to know Emma and Terry well. Each had conveyed to me her thoughts and feelings with such simple candor that I could easily guess what went on inside of them. I had tried to shut out their torment as I usually did during difficult consultations. But now their words clung to me till I realized that the dream of my mother had broken my defense against the sorrow of her death. What I had fought against so many years, the awareness of the grief ordained for all of us, now overwhelmed me.

Terry's serious eyes looked at me and made me flinch. I agreed with her that there was no choice but to place her mother in a rest home. There was no reason, I had told her, for further examination.

Now I realized how cold I must have seemed to Terry and Emma when I had proclaimed what was "best for all concerned." At that time I was unaware of what my pomposity concealed.

But Terry requested that I reexamine her mother this evening following her admission to the home, "just to be certain we're not making a mistake." I agreed reluctantly.

"Poor Violet," a nurse said. "She mumbles all day long, but no one can understand her. Do you think she's trying to say something to us?"

"Say something!" the old head nurse replied. "No! Lands no! 'Ha, tha, tha, tha tha' is all she ever says. Dr. Longman says she has the kind of aphasia that lets her say words, but she doesn't know what they mean. Enough to drive you crazy with her sputtering and mumbling all day and all night long, grabbing for anything that she touches—'grasp reflex' is what they call it. But she really doesn't know anyone or anything."

"Seems such a shame," the other said.

"Well, won't hurt her none now. She's in another world. But tell the aides to be sure to feed her slow. She'll swallow when she gets food in her mouth—if she doesn't choke on it. That's about all she'll do for us. She'll have to be fed intravenously if she starts coughing. And that'll mean more work and more trouble." She took a deep breath or two and slowly leaned her weight behind the medicine cart, which creaked forward hesitantly, followed by a retinue of equally apathetic medical personnel.

"OK, let's start our rounds. Here we go again."

Near the nurse's station sat a man in a wheelchair, his head fallen over onto his chest, spittle dribbling from his mouth, the remains of his morning cream-of-wheat caked on his face.

The practical nurse who attended him sat reading for long, silent periods, occasionally turning to stare blankly at the wall, engrossed in the book she held before her: *Christ and the Last Days of Man.*

"Why the struggle of these inhabitants?" she mumbled to herself, "and whence go we from here?" When the old man groaned she looked up, unseeing, turned her head down and continued to read.

The elderly lay in beds close to each other, two to four in a room, amid a pervasive stench of urine.

The door to Violet's room was open. From my vantage point, I could see without being seen. Violet's room was painted bright by the hot sunlight of the afternoon. A roommate lay silent and motionless, with one arm and leg sticking out above the covers, a thin layer of loose muscle shrouding the skeleton beneath. Her bracelet dangled from what seemed a pencil-thin limb. Only occasional movements of her lips told me she was alive.

Violet sat upright in her chair, mumbling as she gazed out the window, shunning the scene about her. Her arm bore a bracelet inscribed: "Violet Robinson." It was a symbol of the tenuousness of both existence and identity that everyone, the living and the dead, was tagged. Finally Emma entered, hobbling behind a walking chair, a device that provided support as she moved.

I rose and moved closer, carefully remaining out of view, my curiosity still more aroused by what I had gazed at, yet refused to see, these past years: what really took place with my elderly patients when I was absent.

Violet said, "Ha, tha, tha, tha, tha."

I knew by Emma's answer that she thought Violet had asked about her walk. Emma nodded soberly. "I used to walk around the apartment at home every morning to water my plants. There are no plants in this room." Her creased face accumulated new circles around her dull grey eyes when she spoke.

Terry entered. Obedient to her mother's needs, she had walked her and talked with her, spending several hours this first day. Helping her mother into bed, she hurried to depart. With a forced smile, she said, "Goodbye, Mother. Enjoy the fruit. I'll be here next Sunday." She pointed to a package on the bed. With a last look at her mother and a quick kiss on her mother's cheek, Terry departed, closing the door after her.

Terry had told me what she thought whenever she imagined herself closing the door of her mother's room at the Seaside for the first time. "Mother said herself, 'With your small apartment, I couldn't stay with you and Bill—and the children. They're grown up now and need their own rooms—and I'm too weak to live alone again.'"

Despite her words, I knew that Emma was staring silently after her daughter, looking as if she were a child betrayed. She hoped the door would open again.

On the other side, Terry paused, also looking at the door, unmoving until she noticed me. I could see in her darkened face that a childhood memory arose in her as she had predicted to me that it would.

Terry was seven when her only pet, a playful elderly cat, died. Her mother explained again and again, "Dying is just a long, long sleep from which Camille will never awaken," and that was why they had to bury the silent, swollen, white-furred animal in the back yard beneath the sweet-smelling magnolia trees. Then she saw her mother shut her bedroom door. Terry called her back into her room half-a-dozen times.

"But how can my cat breathe in the ground?"

"Death is hard for anyone to understand," her mother finally said, taking and holding one of Terry's hands for a long time.

"Yes," Terry said, weeping, "but I just can't leave her there in the ground, Mother. Don't you see? She'll get wet when it rains."

Terry turned and made a movement toward the door. She paused, spun away abruptly, and left, nodding tearfully to me as she passed.

The nurses had assured Terry that her mother would "get used to it."

Down the hallway the nurses walked more rapidly now. I knew their procedure. It was always the same. The head nurse held a tray of syringes as she entered each room; she matter-of-factly targeted her injections, hardly checking the patient's name card under each syringe against the doctor's order label as she moved from one patient to another.

The ulcerated areas on the buttocks of each patient unable to turn were tended by the second nurse and a silent aide, who laboriously rolled the supine patient onto his abdomen. Yet week after week, month after month, the inevitable bleeding ulcerated areas grew deeper. The second nurse approached each patient with the same fixed smile she wore on her face on Sunday for visitors. The head nurse's face, grown chronically weary and cynical with the years, was a cold mask that she directed at the inhabitants with a disdainful inclination of her head.

I felt my face flush with anger at her and at the utterly painful helplessness of every patient. The inevitable event that I always beheld with dread now took shape brightly before my eyes, removed from the twilight of my repression. As I became aware of the rage in myself I realized that anger was the reactive barrier I habitually erected to shield me from despair whenever my repression failed.

Now the head nurse approached Emma's room. I walked away as if moving on, then returned unnoticed to my former position. The emaciated woman winced when she received her shot, then opened her eyes again to stare into space at nothing. Emma, now weeping silently inside herself, clutched an embroidered handkerchief she had made a long time ago while her small daughter had watched with wonderment. It matched the hand-sewn pink-and-yellow bedspreads and pillow cases and embroidery that had adorned her little home long after her husband had passed away. These sewn pieces were now at her daughter's apartment, neatly packed away in boxes except for a blanket and some handkerchiefs that she had brought with her to her new home. She had tried to encourage her daughter by saying, "Keep my furniture for just a little while, till maybe I can get stronger and have my own apartment again."

The head nurse, taking a long, slow breath, approached Emma. Emma saw the large white pill in the nurse's hand. Her pupils grew frozen, her mouth fell open and fixed.

"This is for you to take," the head nurse said.

"What is it?"

"Your doctor ordered it for bedtime."

"But I can sleep all right."

"Now, please don't argue. Your doctor ordered it for you, in case you need it."

"But I can sleep all right."

"You look upset to me. Take it. It should help you sleep."

Emma's eyes turned down and she swallowed the pill.

"They make you take all sorts of medicines you don't need," she had tearfully predicted despite my reassurances.

Was she thinking of the time when Terry was seven years old and developed a deep-red rash over her abdomen? A robust, coarse-skinned neighbor woman poured a black liquid from a medicine bottle she held in her hand. "It will be good for the child," the intruder had insisted. "It'll stop the fever that's bound to come."

Emma was uncertain, but she knew how expensive doctors were. She watched her frightened daughter as the woman pushed a spoonful of tar-smelling liquid into Terry's mouth and forced her to swallow.

The head nurse stared at Emma, who reached across to the next bed to take Violet's hand. Violet grasped the unexpected hand and turned toward Emma with what Emma knew was a reassuring look.

"Thank you," Emma said to Violet. "I've never lived away from home before except when we went to my cousin's wedding in Iowa. This all seems so strange to me."

I could see my mother lying in her bed one late night when I visited the Seaside unexpectedly. A stern night-shift aide was speaking to her. "Please, don't press the nursing light again for help tonight. That's the third time you've called me. What's wrong now? You can feed yourself."

I wanted to plunge into the room, grab the head nurse by the throat, and tell her that neither the physician in charge nor I intended that Emma should be forced to take a sleeping pill or anything else.

I could have torn the nurse apart in my fury and enjoyed it. It would have been a pleasure to attack her; my face was burning with it.

The head nurse now spoke to Emma. "With all them elderly people in the other beds to be concerned about, we can't be called back all the time worrying about people who can't sleep," she said. "If a doctor won't order a sleeping pill a patient needs, I give it to him anyway, or I just refuse to take care of that patient. That's all."

The second nurse smiled and nodded.

Violet, muttering, was being fed. She gasped and began to choke.

"Feed her nice and slow," the head nurse admonished her aide. "I told you, you have to be careful."

"I can help feed her, long as I'm here in the room with her," Emma offered, "if I can get my walking chair close enough."

"Maybe," the head nurse said, looking at Emma. Then her nostrils dilated with sniffing and a scowl crossed her face.

Emma felt the moisture of her B.M. before she could control it. This had occurred with increasing frequency in the past few months. The corners of her mouth were pulled down, but she was too bewildered to cry. The nurses and their aide brusquely changed her sheets and clothing.

Was Emma thinking of her little daughter with the cat, and how Terry wet herself during the night of its death? Emma reassured her weeping, embarrassed daughter while she helped her change her clothing.

I was a young child. How old? Eight or nine? My mother was caring for me as I lay in my darkened room terrified by spasms of coughing and wheezing from the pneumonia that cut my breath off. Was I dying? I heard the doctor whisper to my mother.

"If you can afford a hospital, your boy would have nursing care around the clock," the doctor said. "That's the only advantage of hospitalization. You could get some rest." There was an oxygen tank in my room already.

I remained at home. My mother never left my side for more than a few moments over the next few weeks till my fever broke.

The nurses finished wiping and dressing Emma. The head nurse's face was taut.

"In a real hospital, the charge nurses don't have to give medications and help with this too," she said to the second nurse.

The aide placed the smeared sheets in the hamper and wheeled it out.

Emma heard the nurse's words. She felt her face flush as she grew dizzy. She closed her eyes. I guessed what visions might come to her. When she opened them, she saw the distorted face of her small infant daughter sitting in bed toothless and grinning. Then it grew into another face with raw and boneless gums. It was Violet, opening and closing her jaws, chewing a remnant of a past meal. Then Violet pulled at the ends of her sheets, put them into her mouth, and began to suck them.

Outside, the nurse asked her aide for the daily census.

The aide replied in a tiny voice, "Forty-six women, thirty-eight men, ma'am."

"Thirty-nine," she corrected her aide.

"No, thirty-eight since this morning, ma'am."

"Oh yes," the head nurse said, "that old Mr. Alfred in the corner of 221. The one who kept squirming out of his chair. He never could sit comfortable anywhere in or out of bed. Yes. Now I remember."

Emma stared at the door again. Violet grunted some sounds. Again I sensed what was taking place. Emma thought she heard Violet try to repeat Terry's parting words, "She'll be back again, dear. Your daughter will be back on Sunday."

Emma wept openly now. She reached across and held Violet's hand again. Violet's hand clamped shut and the two women lay that way for a while. Then Emma fell asleep and, I imagined, dreamt: Terry was a small girl playing with a white kitten, while Emma—vigorous, young, and smiling—watched her.

In a few moments my rage disappeared like some savage fire that burned fiercely for a moment, then lay extinguished in a crumpled heap of ashes. A sense of despair crept back and took hold of me. I saw my mother's face again. But now my repression would no longer take over and keep me from this feeling. The anguish of my elderly patient clung to me like Violet's grasp and refused to let go.

Chapter 10
Howard and Bruce and the Children Sweet

And the children! The children are the source and the pituitary of my continuation and my future pleasure. In them I see my history, how it was and how I should have liked it to be. Am I not a child still, the kernels of my past growing within me, within my unconscious, layered over by decades of neocortical life, disguised by the mantle of adulthood? And when I regress in anguish, anger, humiliation, or joy, I see the child in myself once more; my past is still alive. Yes, my immortality may be trod upon by the years, but never buried, even by death, if some child influenced by me lives on after me; every child I touch takes a bit of me with him.

Their little lives unfold; their futures develop before my eyes. Then I wonder what becomes of them in later years, till I see them in every adult who appears before me.

Daily over a period of many months, I stood unobtrusively in some corner of the play-yard or classroom observing the nursery children as they arrived to spend the morning. Sometimes I joined them in their activities. This was part of my training.

As I watched, I wondered over and over again about the multiple forces that shaped and directed them from their earliest years on, granted that even infants differ widely from each other from the moment of birth. Some—those I had seen before anyone else on earth as I delivered them slithering and moist from their brief maternal journey—cried with clenched fists in red-faced rage that they should be forced to begin their extrauterine life on earth; others slept in yawning contentment, placid from their first moment on, till caused to cry by the errant hand that delivered them.

Slowly, singly, some children arrived at the small nursery school clinging to their parents' hands, whining and crying as a father or mother pushed them through the gate. Others came smiling and gleeful with chatter and expected playful pleasures, running and shouting in a chorus of excited anticipation. The play-yard resounded with what seemed to be a hundred voices, though there were only a few dozen children.

Having seen me about so frequently, the group of mothers and children regarded me as just another of the friendly adults in the nursery and appeared to be quite at ease in my presence.

"Look how sweetly the children come to play all morning," Howard's mother said to Nene's as she dropped her son off in the play-yard.

"To be a child again," Howard's mother continued. She kissed her boy goodbye and said, "Have fun, Howard."

He shouted affectionately, "Good-bye, you booby," and waved to her.

Nene's mother nodded her head, but only mechanically, in response to the other woman. She dropped her daughter off hurriedly with a mumbled word or two, and without a good-bye. Nene, without turning to wave or talk to her mother, entered the yard and sat by herself as usual till one teacher said, "Come over here and join us—we're having fun."

"Lemme alone," Bruce said to his mother as he shrugged off her hug.

"He's mean in the morning, just like his daddy," Bruce's mother said aloud to anyone who would listen. "I guess all men are alike, especially in the morning—it's hard to get to like them."

The children played outdoors for an hour as usual when they first arrived.

"Juice time," a teacher yelled, smiling.

"Yay! Yay! Yay!" the children shouted in a deafening chorus. Into the classroom they rushed.

During the juice period and afterward, the teacher read a story. A large group of children sat on a rug on the floor with the teacher facing them. Howard and Bruce sat by themselves across the room, having stealthily carried off some crackers and bananas.

Howard said, "This is a very nice lunch." He took the pitcher and spilled more juice for Bruce.

Then Howard said, "Here are more bananas."

Bruce replied, "Oh yes, you live in a banana house." With that both five-year-old boys laughed suddenly, uproariously, obscenely, the unconscious portent of their mirth shaking them irreverently. They continued to talk to each other, and Bruce told Howard about a stray dog he had to give away because it yelped too much at night. Howard informed Bruce, "You must always keep a dog on a leash and have a dog house for it." He was quite vehement.

Bruce said, "But make sure the dog knows you're the boss. Sometimes you have to whip it."

As the story was being read, Bruce continued to speak in a low voice. "Get some more crackers from the cracker box behind her. It's in the corner." Then they whispered frantically to each other. Bruce finally said, "Yeah, that's the way."

Howard went up to the teacher and said, "Can I get a drink of water?" Before she could answer yes he slithered halfway across the room, sneaked some crackers, and brought them back into the corner. The teacher pretended to be unaware and continued reading. Both boys ate with the gusto of starving heathens.

Howard was extremely large, with a round, full face, wrinkled jowls, and big, black, mirthful eyes. His voice was gruff and deep, his pants baggy, his shirt wrinkled and dirty so that he more closely resembled a husky Hollywood henchman than a boy not quite six years of age. Bruce, the smaller of the two, had a narrow forehead that often wrinkled into a frown, his face seeming old and wizened. When Howard accidentally bumped into a classmate, the child laughed and stuck an elbow into the friendly buffoon, who laughed in return. When Bruce approached another child out of sight of the teacher, Bruce clenched his teeth, snarling or threatening with a fist, while the child shrank from him with a scream or slunk away in silence. At those moments I felt my anger rise toward Bruce.

It was unreasonable, even unconscionable, for me to feel antipathy toward a small boy whom I hardly knew. I felt ashamed of it. From the first day of my observations, I could detect that Bruce was a child who was universally disliked except by Howard, the only one big enough to appear to be unafraid of him.

These two boys' dominant positions were well established among the children of the nursery.

As the two sat alone at a small table in the darkest corner of the room, gesturing and speaking in hushed tones, they resembled two thieves in the night huddled beneath a candle-lit table in one of Hollywood's shadowy little coffee houses.

The teacher, lifting her head to look at them, said, "As long as you two are not ready for a story, you may sit together where you are, but you must be quiet." They guffawed at her remarks and continued as if engaged in some clandestine proposition as they hunched over their table, half-hidden objects spread before them, now alternately talking in gruff, hoarse voices or intense, secret whispers.

At one point Howard unexpectedly left Bruce and sat down to catch part of the story. Nene, who sat alone nearby, protested in an irritated tone, "I can't see." Howard moved aside, inadvertently resting on her leg. Nene struggled to get her foot from beneath his hulking frame. The class giggled.

When the story was over, the teacher asked whose turn it was to call the names for the children to leave the group one at a time to play again.

"Gigi," the children shouted.

Gigi called Howard's name first. Howard got up, walked over to her, kissed her on the cheek, and went off joyously as the children laughed. Gigi shrank back, smiled, and called the next name. "Debbie, and no kissing please. He's always doing that."

The children waited their turns, and one by one they were called. Nene, sitting alone, was the last to be summoned.

Bruce said, "Tomorrow is my turn to call names."

Howard responded in a loud voice, looking at the teacher, "Yeah, tomorrow is his turn." Howard and Bruce went off and continued to play together.

Bruce said, "I'm the strong man."

Howard affirmed, "Yeah, he's the strong man."

Howard found a toy house and put it in the middle of a small table. "There's water coming in the house. It's drownding the people." The two began to play earnestly again. Howard continued, "The people in the house are dead and they gotta have help to make them better." He dragged the table over to Bruce and began to take small dolls out of the house, handing them to Bruce. Bruce placed them on a low table beside the house.

Howard said, "There's father; he's all right."

"Yeah," said Bruce, "and here's brother; he's OK too. He's squeezed dry."

Howard added, "Mother's OK and so is the baby."

Bruce retorted unexpectedly, a flash of anger in his face, "Naw, mother's dead!" And with that declaration he kicked the house and left the game. "Don't get in my way, Nene," he challenged, crossing in front of her. Then he deliberately thrust his face close to hers, a defiant rage in his eyes.

The frightened girl hesitated and spluttered, "Well?" as if to question his next move.

Again, Bruce insolently stuck his face in front of Nene and volleyed forth a mocking, "Well, well, well, well!"

"Don't do that!" she said, shrinking away.

"Don't do that!" Bruce mimicked, dancing toward her, his angular white face intent and seemingly too brutal for a child.

Howard watched.

Bruce bumped into her. "Nene's dead," he laughed. "She's drownded in the house."

Howard laughed, too, a conciliatory ring in his voice. "Nene's dead." He tried to get Nene to laugh also.

Bruce bumped her again and barked a jeering laugh into her face.

Nene's fragile body slumped to the floor. She wilted under the horrendous attack. An outburst of pitiful crying shook her. She lay there, alone; she had no intrapsychic object to console her. The blows cut deeply into her and touched the painful indifference with which she was regarded by her mother. I knew. I had been observing the woman these past few months.

A wave of hurt and anger came upon me. I'll step in and crack the boy's skull. The damned teachers are elsewhere, preoccupied with trivia. They're permitting the murder of a soul.

Then I paused. No. I must let it go on. It was my job to learn, I argued with myself, my teeth clenched—to learn about the emotional development of children and their society, not to intervene.

Howard observed Nene. His smile was gone. Bruce threw the mother doll from the house. He stepped on her and said, "That's Nene." He ground the heel of his foot into the doll. Now he approached Nene menacingly.

I felt the full fury of nearly six years of hatred stored up in him, in his arrogant childish smile. Suddenly I re-experienced a scene that took place when I was a small child during which I was as humiliated and terrorized as Nene at this moment. Now I knew why I felt so strongly. I had grown furious at him, at a child who was attacking me in effigy, attacking a part of me that once existed. I wanted to kill him.

Howard balked, picking up the house. "They're getting better," he insisted. He picked up the dolls from the table, one by one. Finally he paused. The mother doll remained on the floor. Several children were now staring silently, alert to the significance of the scene.

"She's better too," Howard said, picking up the crushed doll from the floor and interposing himself between Bruce and Nene, who had moved away.

"She's dead!" Bruce insisted, taking a step toward Nene.

"But she's got better," Howard said again, replacing the doll in the house. "I got her better," and clumsily he strode between Nene and Bruce, brushing against Bruce.

Bruce pushed Howard hard. Howard rocked backward. Bruce approached him again and Howard stepped back. Bruce grabbed the fragmented doll and crushed it in his hands. Then he moved toward Nene once more and smashed the doll on the floor. Again Howard's huge hulk came between them. Bruce shoved him. This time Howard moved back only slightly.

Bruce scowled, but the massive child stood fast and said in a voice half-pleading, half-threatening, "Let's play something else."

Bruce turned and walked away. A sense of frustrated rage burned red on his cheeks. Howard watched Nene as she staggered, frightened and silent, across the classroom and sat down alone as usual.

Chapter 11
Myrna the
Lonely One

"She picked up a sharp knife and rushed at the baby. Imagine, her own nephew, a three-month-old baby!" Myrna's mother wailed. "First time my son had brought our grandchild over to our house. Then she ran toward me with the knife, and then she ran downstairs and said she was going to kill herself—she held it right under her throat. We were so terribly frightened!"

"Her brother and I grabbed her, and we called Dr. Barrington," Myrna's father said in a broken voice.

He appeared to be dapper and vigorous—an architect. I'd heard of him before. She looked much older (though they were both in their early fifties), moderately obese, worn, an "old" grey, immobile in her chair.

They continued telling me about Myrna and the events leading to her admission.

"She was always a tense and delicate child, even as a little girl of two or three," her mother said in a husky, imploring tone. "But she never was difficult till these last five or six years. She's twenty-five now. These last few years, she's become terribly suspicious and stubborn—always seems so angry, and always says that I care for her brother, Leslie, more than I do for her. That isn't true. It simply isn't—"

"She and her mother have always been too damned close her whole life," Myrna's father interrupted. "Always acted as if her mother were going to disappear and never come back. She wouldn't let her out of sight ever since she was a baby."

"Yes," Mrs. McFadden agreed. "She was always very dependent on me, especially now. I'll never forget her hysterics when her father and I went away overnight once, when she was about nine or ten. Up to then, we rarely left her. The housekeeper called us in Balboa and said, 'Myrna's driving me insane. She's so worried about you, Mrs. McFadden. She's frantic, crying, and carrying on so for the last six hours. I just had to call you! Most kids will stop after a while, but she isn't about to. She thinks you'll never come back because you're sick or hurt—or something! I can't figure her out, but you've just got to come home right now!'

"That was in the days," Mrs. McFadden continued, "when her father and I went out together once in a while." She looked at her husband.

He failed to look back at her. "As I was saying," Mr. McFadden said, "she and her mother always have had a thing going between 'em. They're inseparable."

"Not that I wanted it that way," Mrs. McFadden said. "You were just never around to see her much. Even when she was real young you were awfully busy all the time. I had to take care of both kids by myself."

"No use going over that again now," he said. "At this moment we have Myrna to worry about."

"But the doctor was just asking me about Myrna's childhood! You have to understand, doctor," she said, turning to me again. "I never wanted Myrna to depend on me so much, but—well, I guess I was the only one she could talk with and I suppose because I was lonely and troubled, she felt it. I don't mean her father didn't care; he always was concerned about her. But he just never saw her much—had to travel a lot, and even when he was in the city he always came home late." She stopped to look at him again.

He sat quietly, rubbing his neck. She glanced at him several times as she spoke.

Her pleading seemed painful (or was it only a remnant of what had once contained pain?). She was revealing her loss of him as a husband and father. Now in this crisis was she making one last attempt to force him to recant? No chance! He felt no remorse for her.

Was there a sadness in her? No. More of a flatness of affect, as if she had given up long ago. She seemed distant, as if part of her were elsewhere. She, too, must be part of Myrna's treatment. I suspected that Myrna felt that she and her mother had merged into one and were indistinguishable from each other. I knew that I must talk with Myrna's mother alone in the next day or so.

"She really was a strange little child," Mr. McFadden said. "Never seemed to play with dolls or toys like other little girls, never laughed or had much fun. Just followed her mother around from room to room. Wouldn't even let her mother sit on the toilet without pounding on the door and screaming to get in. She never had any playmates the way our son Leslie did. I remember because her kindergarten teacher once called us for a special conference. Said she had to talk to both of us. She pointed out that Myrna related to no one, that she was an unusual child. She just walked back and forth in the yard, wouldn't sit down and paint or play or be part of the group in any way, although she was very bright and learned fast. She wasn't surprised when I told her that Myrna refused to go to nursery school."

"When I tried for months to take her to preschool," Mrs. McFadden said, "she screamed and made such a fuss that I never could keep her there. She seemed to be in such a fright when I left her, the nursery teacher said, and I agreed with her. Why make a child suffer?"

Mr. McFadden said, "I told the kindergarten teacher that whenever I tried to put her on my lap to play with her, even before she could walk, she just squirmed off and would have no part of me. When she was older, I could rarely get her to talk to me. She wasn't ever interested, and I guess I gave up trying.

"I suppose I need affection, too, and when she didn't want to come to me, my feelings were hurt. Sounds strange to me now—my feelings being hurt by a baby.

"Her second-grade teacher recommended we talk to our pediatrician. He wasn't modern, didn't believe in all those 'emotional problems.' All he said was, 'She'll grow out of it. Put her in a private school if those public school teachers can't handle her.' Some friends said we should see another pediatrician, but I guess I didn't want to bother so I told them I was following the advice of a doctor I respected. Maybe all this wouldn't have happened if we had gotten some help for her then."

I left the visitors' room and went onto the psychiatry ward to meet Myrna.

She was slender, almost thin. Her blue eyes were fixed in a bewildered stare. Her face would have been attractive if it weren't pinched with terror.

I saw a nurse speak my name to her. She raced toward me. "Let me out of here! Let me out! Let me go home! You're keeping me here because you think I killed someone! There's gas coming in through those pipes in the walls—gas—what are they trying to do to me?" She ran toward a window and pushed hard against the screen. The heavy mesh held tight. She pounded her fist against it several times, stopped, and walked back slowly.

"Please, I want my mother. She needs me, don't you see? She can't be without me. She has to have me. Please, let me go before they kill her too!"

I felt her anguish as it swept across her face and filled the room.

"Why are you keeping me here? Who are you?"

I said, "I'm Dr. Sherwood. Dr. Barrington asked me to see you."

Her eyes fixed on me and refused to move.

She suspected me too. In her expressions I saw her sudden changes and contradictions of mood and thought.

During that moment, I could see again the severely manic young woman I saw years ago at a state hospital. I was making morning ward rounds in the acute intensive treatment unit. This was her first day in the hospital. The moment I entered the small isolation unit on which she was kept, she sprang toward me, flailing at my face with nails as long as an animal's claws (why weren't they cut?). She gashed my left cheek, narrowly missing my eye. Two female attendants ran toward her. She darted away from them and climbed the screen of her isolation unit like a tigress in a cage.

"Who would want to harm your mother?"

"She needs me," she said, ignoring my words. "My mother needs me. But why am I here? I haven't done anything." She began to weep suddenly. "Oh no! They've probably killed her already, these people." She motioned toward some patients in the hospital corridor. "They've already killed my mother!"

I waited, then spoke carefully. "Your mother is safe, Myrna. And you're safe too, here in the hospital. No one, no matter how he or she feels, will be allowed to harm either of you."

"Come, dear," a nurse said, leading Myrna back to her room. I looked at my childlike patient as she hesitantly moved away. She glanced back at me.

Terror, the sheer terror in her face! It was a nightmare that refused to disappear even after she was awake. What devastating experience caused her to react this way? It was my guess that she needed reassurance which would make her feel protected from destruction and from her own destructiveness toward others. Her defensive paranoid reactions were generated from fear and a resultant rage, which she projected onto others. It was usually this way with patients with her kind of illness. I hoped that the safety of the hospital would soon reassure her from her horror. This was an acute episode.

My immediate course of action was to try to restore Myrna to her pre-psychotic state and to help her gain control of the gyrating affect that now commanded her thought processes. I ordered chlorpromazine, a psychiatric drug, in large amounts, as well as other drugs and constant nursing care.

Then I asked her mother to meet with me alone in my private office two days later.

"He was never home when the children were small," Myrna's mother said slowly, her face expressionless. Even her clothing, though new and neatly tailored, appeared on her to be faded and colorless. "Gone nearly every night to a meeting or something. Of course, I understand a young architect getting started has lots of things to do. But it was always that way, from the time Myrna was born. He never had much time for me, either. His parents had money and they gave him everything, and I guess he just got used to having things his own way."

"What things do you mean?"

She hesitated before speaking. "I suppose a man needs the companionship of his wife, but once the children come she's tied up. And I guess there just was too much to do around a big house like ours. And I'd get so tired all the time." Her chair creaked as she shifted.

"Then, too, soon after Myrna was born I began to develop those awful headaches and 'funny spells.' I'd become fuzzy-headed and have to lie down all the time. None of the doctors seemed to know what they were. I still have those spells, even now, and I have to take all kinds of medicines."

She still avoided what she had started to tell me. I decided not to press her on this now. But for the next hour I prodded her to tell me in great detail of her illness and of Myrna's infancy and childhood. Then I asked her to return to the waiting room while I spoke with Mr. McFadden.

"Right after Myrna was born her mother became different," Myrna's father said. He looked directly at me with dark, intense eyes. "It was an unmistakable change. She said she wanted children, yet she never appeared enthusiastic about them. She felt she didn't really know how to take care of infants, though we had a housekeeper, and a cook, and anyone else she wanted to help her. She never seemed to enjoy them as babies—you know, how some women coo and play with little ones. Oh yes, she saw to it that they were properly fed and clothed and clean all those years, but I knew there was something else missing, some kind of—I don't know how to put it, other than some kind of pleasure. They always seemed to be such a terrible burden to her.

"From the beginning Myrna craved so much more attention than Leslie. He's two years younger. Maybe because he was a boy, or maybe because he got more from his mother. I dont't know. Myrna was such a clinging, scared child. She wouldn't let her mother out of her sight. Then right after she was born, Mrs. McFadden began having those damned headaches and dizziness. None of the doctors could find anything to explain them, but she had to hole up in her room all day long and take pills and sleep while the maids took care of the baby. Seems as if life was just too much for her. One doctor kept giving her Demerol and Seconal for headaches for years. She claimed she had to have them.

"Those children just didn't have much of their mother. Even when she was with them she just sat in one chair all day long like a zombie while they crawled around. But Myrna still kept one eye on her mother. I could understand boys, somehow, a little more than girls, so I spent some time with Leslie, though I'm not much with children either."

Zombie! I saw what he meant. Some doctors write as many prescriptions for drugs as a patient wants, as if these doctors don't give a damn.

"By the time she was three, Myrna still wouldn't come to me or anyone else except her mother. We couldn't even send her to nursery school because when we tried, she cried all day and night and carried on so, she didn't sleep for a week. The teachers said they'd better not have her till she was four or five. But even then she wouldn't go.

"Probably her mother's crazy sicknesses all the time had a lot to do with it, because when Myrna was only maybe four or five she started worrying not just about her mother's going away but about her mother's getting sick or dying. She fretted about all the doctors her mother saw, and why her mother got all those shots, and why her mother looked so sick all the time, and why her mother always had a headache, and why her mother had to go away even for an hour or two, and if she didn't come back right away, did something happen to her, was she in an accident or was she dead?—and on and on and on. This went on for years.

"Finally a consultant said, 'Headaches or not, Mrs. McFadden can't take Demerol and Seconal anymore! She's addicted!' We had to put her in the hospital for two months to get her off everything. And poor Myrna, she was so panicked about her mother, she tore around the house day and night in a fidget. She couldn't sleep and couldn't eat the whole time, though everyone kept telling her that her mother was all right. Myrna lost so much weight she became a sickly skeleton. Her pediatrician was ready to hospitalize her too. Finally I just had to sneak Myrna onto the ward against the rules to see her mother. What a terrible scene that was! Myrna grabbed her mother and clung so desperately, she left five bleeding fingernail marks in both her mother's arms. The nurses had to pry her loose so I could take her home.

"But even after Mrs. McFadden came home she began to go around secretly getting prescriptions from other doctors—sleeping pills and what not—all over again.

"No man can live with that kind of wife. I admit I haven't been the best of fathers, but I just couldn't take it." Tears came to his eyes, but he still sat upright, looking at me with no attempt to avert his symmetrical, impressive face.

Again, Myrna's mother and I were alone.

"When I was pregnant with Myrna a friend of mine told me that people had seen my husband out with some of the cocktail waitresses from the Golden Bull." Her voice quavered. "I wouldn't believe her at first.

"I guess I could never quarrel with him. I'm just not the type. I stayed with him for the children's sake because I was ill—those fuzzy spells with the terrible headaches—I didn't want the children to be alone with just a sick mother to care for them. I just loved them too much to do that. If I'd been well I would have left him long ago. But no one, none of the doctors, seemed to be able to do anything to help me . . ."

Myrna sat in the corner of her room when I entered. It was the third day. She was staring out the window when my footsteps startled her.

"I've got to go home," she cried. "My mother—she's dead—and she needs me to bury her—to bury her—in the sand." She wrung her hands and began to weep. "She needs me—to put her to rest."

Myrna's delusions were expressions of her unconscious conflicts. The infant nephew had threatened her overwhelming need for exclusive possession of her mother. Her mother, "killed by others," freed the patient of her anger and her guilt for her murderous impulses. Now her mother would no longer be able to render affection to another. Was the ambivalent aspect of Myrna's wish shown by her genuine grief and sorrow over her "mother's death"? In fact, Myrna's own throat had been lacerated superficially by the sharp edge of the knife the moment before it had been wrested from her. Was that Myrna's expiation for the sinful wish to kill her mother? To bury mother also had significance. Myrna and mother often played a game of "bury mother in the sand" at the beach during Myrna's early childhood, one of the few pleasurable private times she had with her mother before her brother's birth intervened. Mother enjoyed falling asleep on a hot summer's day while her little daughter busily played with a shovel, digging and pouring the cool sand on mother's limbs and body, leaving only her head exposed.

I now had a few clues as to why Myrna was undergoing a psychotic episode. But some areas of the jigsaw puzzle were still missing. What was the nature of the intimate transactions with her mother? Myrna had had deep-rooted emotional conflicts since early childhood. How did they influence her fundamental ego development? Would her ego integrative capacities be sufficient to halt her present psychotic regression, or would her downhill course continue and become irreversible?

I felt a sudden oppression, a constriction in my throat and chest— somatized anxiety on my part. My thoughts drifted back many years to a period of training I had had at a large psychiatric state hospital.

Section "G" of Milford Hospital was full of women, most grey-haired and pale, sitting impassively upon rows of wooden benches on the musty wards and silent corridors. They stared at the floor or into space. Some shielded their eyes from the sunlight that pierced the windows, a persistent, startling intruder which focused on the scene and revealed it to the world. Yet there was no one but the patients to view it, save an occasional nurse's aide passing through. The slow, monotonous beat of the old wall clock at the end of the hall reinforced the absence of change. Life seemed suspended under the silence-breaking staccato of the timepiece.

"Come, dear," a kind matron named Amy said, leading a thin, bewildered-looking creature back to her ward. The patient held the matron's hand with reluctant trust. It had been fourteen years since Bernice had come on the ward. She would take no other hand but Amy's. Most of the day, Bernice sat on the floor, twirling herself in restless, tireless circles, fingering her nose, her mouth, her anus, her ears, her vaginal orifice, involved entirely with her body and her own inner world except when she was led to her tray to be fed or to the fenced compound to be aired.

This ward of the hospital was unique, even for the custodial care sections. For on section "G" the most regressed women were contained. Bernice wore no dress or ordinary garb, but a sacklike gown over diapers or no undergarment at all. Here she lived, tended by her keepers very much like an animal in a zoo. The men had their counterpart on the other side of the hospital.

At noon, if the sun was warm, a strange procession of antediluvianlike people, perhaps three hundred in all, were led outside.

The quiet patients, like herded beasts, arranged themselves in a disheveled, shuffling row as they moved into the assigned area—the catatonics, most mute of all, soon to assume their characteristic frozen poses.

Agitated patients were not allowed on this ward, but occasionally a chronically withdrawn patient emerged into a wild, gesticulating dance, sometimes attacking, more likely dashing from an imagined oppressor.

Bernice's family history and her age had been strikingly similar to Myrna's when she entered the hospital fourteen years before. Bernice remained in the hospital after I left, and probably will be there forever.

If I made a serious error in diagnosis or treatment, Myrna could spend years, even the rest of her life, in a psychiatric hospital. This might happen anyway, no matter what I did.

Tomorrow was the seventh day, I thought. I'll risk a meeting between Myrna and her mother. If Myrna can be reassured by seeing her mother alive, it means that she is recovering and that the forces of reality are taking over. Seeing her mother would then be therapeutic for her. But if Myrna saw her mother and reacted with stress, it could be damaging to Myrna's recovery and possibly cause her psychosis to deepen.

Mrs. McFadden entered the visitors' room with a grim look. Myrna stared at her.

"I've come to visit you, Myrna dear," she said.

Myrna covered her eyes with her arms, turned away, and shook her head. Then she whirled about and screamed, "Who are you? Get out of here! My God! Get out of here! My mother's dead!" She stamped her feet in an angry, strange dance, then began to sob loudly and dashed out the door back to her room.

Damn! So that's how it was! Life's still too much for my patient. I had done all I could be expected to do. Why should I condemn myself or hold myself responsible if she failed to recover? What more could any other psychiatrist do? I must look at my feeling of rising despair and my dread of failure.

It was nearly ten, time for the morning staff meeting. Maybe someone, including the full-time staff psychiatrists, would have some ideas. I could use consultation.

My throat and chest felt even more taut as I took Myrna's chart from the rack in the nurses' station. Another startling event came to my attention. The nursing notes indicated that Myrna had eaten no breakfast that morning. Nor had she eaten much supper the night before.

"She said she wasn't very hungry each time," Mrs. Roe stated at the staff meeting. She was a skilled nurse with a plain but kind face. "Myrna's weight has dropped eight or ten pounds since admission."

"She didn't eat much even on the day she came in," an aide pointed out.

After the meeting I returned to the ward. Myrna sat apart from the rest of the patients in the dayroom. She gazed at me with a frozen, frightened look. As I approached, she shrank away.

"Come with the doctor, please," Mrs. Roe said. Myrna remained. Mrs. Roe took her gently by the hand. "Dr. Sherwood's waiting for you." Myrna pulled her hand free. Another nurse stepped forward and was about to grab her.

"Myrna, please come," I said. Myrna, looking trapped, slowly arose and accompanied me to an interview room on the ward.

"Myrna, you're losing weight. You haven't been eating."

"I can't eat."

"Why not?"

"I can't eat."

The nursing staff had told me that all her vital signs were within normal limits. Her admission physical examination and history had been negative.

"Something is troubling you about the food."

Myrna looked away. "I can't eat."

"You're afraid, aren't you?"

"The people here. They hate me! I know they do." She looked intently at the nurses.

"Myrna—," I began.

"I just know it!"

"You've done nothing to make them dislike you. Why are you afraid of them?"

"There's something wrong with the food. It's not good. There's something in it. When you're not here they put something in it."

"You feel people are trying to do something to you, the same as you feel they are doing to your mother?"

"I know they are," she said, staring at me again. She turned to leave.

"Please stay here, Myrna." I called on the nurses to bring in some cold applesauce and bread, a favorite dessert of Myrna's. Her mother had told me.

"Your own doubts are what make you feel the way you do about the food," I said. A nurse offered her a spoonful. Her eyes widened. She started for the door. Mrs. Roe caught her.

"Let me go! Let me go! Help!" Myrna shrieked. "They're trying to poison me! God—my God, help me! Somebody help me!" She darted out of the room, fighting, screaming, and clawing.

"Ouch!" She had bitten a burly male aide. The nurses pulled Myrna into a seclusion room, her arms flailing. I entered.

"Mrs. Roe will feed you, if you want," I said.

Mrs. Roe approached her. Myrna struck at the spoonful of applesauce. The spoon clanged on the floor. "Take it away—it's poisoned!"

I felt the constrictor muscles tightening again in my chest.

"It's your own fear of poisoning someone and of being poisoned in return for your bad thoughts that worries you, Myrna. But you haven't killed your mother or anyone else. Your thoughts haven't harmed her."

I knew that most of what I said would be rejected now, but I hoped that she would remember my words.

She was given an extra dose of chlorpromazine intramuscularly.

She grew drowsy but still refused to eat. Now I held out a spoonful of applesauce to her. She pretended to nibble at it.

"They fixed it—I still can't eat it!"

I asked to be alone with her. I continued to try to feed her. She turned her face away and moved into a corner of the room. Throughout the next day she touched no food.

"She still won't eat," Mrs. Roe said the following morning. A chill gripped my face and arms. I remembered a male patient at the veterans' hospital years ago. He was treated by a ward psychiatrist under my supervision. The young man had lost more than half his body weight over a period of a year. He had constantly fought his intravenous and gastric-tube feedings despite restraints. He looked like a victim of a Nazi concentration camp, a skeleton kept alive by continual forced feedings. I knew that he ultimately died of malnutrition. No form of treatment, not even electroshock, could alter his belief that his food was poisoned.

I ordered her to be tube-fed at once. It was best to be decisive and to show her I was in control. Her diet would consist of a high grade of liquid protein containing added necessary supplements.

I carefully explained the procedure to Myrna. A tube would be passed through one of her nostrils, down her throat, and into her stomach. Myrna was held tightly by the nurses and attendants. To sedate Myrna more heavily at this moment would be dangerous, for such sedation would diminish or eliminate her gag and cough reflexes and increase the possibility of aspiration of food into her lungs if she should vomit, voluntarily or involuntarily. I decided that I should pass the first tube. What trust I hoped she might develop in me would be extended to the expert technicians and nurses who would repeat the procedure for subsequent meals. The tube was to be withdrawn after each feeding. She struggled to free herself while I quickly passed the tube. Then I placed a large syringe on the open end of the tube, sucking up gastric contents to be certain the tube was in her stomach. The fluid food was injected by the syringe. It flowed slowly down the tube till a pint was in her stomach. Myrna gasped and a deep, guttural belch arose. She pushed her fingers down her throat and tried to vomit. The nurses pounced on her.

"You may be angry, Myrna, but I have to feed you till you decide to eat."

She retched again and again, trying to vomit, while the nurses held her hands.

"Cut it out, damn it!" I heard myself say loudly. "You, Myrna, cut that out right now!"

I felt angry at myself for having to do this to my helpless and weakened patient. I knew what a terrible threat forced feeding was to her. Was I punishing her for frustrating me? I did feel irritated at her for getting worse. Yet I had little choice. Failing to feed her increased the risk of malnutrition. Force-feeding intensified her fear that we were trying to kill her.

I hoped that some observing part of her ego recognized that I wanted her to live and that it was impossible for me to permit her to inflict on herself the punishment of death by starvation. I knew her ambivalence. She wanted to die, yet she was afraid of being killed. How could I reach her to let her know I could be trusted?

I now debated with myself over the use of electroshock therapy, which I had occasionally utilized successfully with other psychotic patients. To startle the brain and body of a person with electroconvulsive seizures always troubled me.

The recent medical literature had reported fair success with some schizophrenic patients using extremely large doses of some of the latest anti-psychotic drugs in addition to chlorpromazine. I decided to give Myrna a four- to six-week trial on these drugs, combined with the intensive ward care and psychotherapy already instituted. If she failed to improve, I would then start electroshock. The longer the psychosis persisted, the less likely she was to emerge.

I explained the gravity of our problem and my treatment plans to Myrna's parents, who indicated their willingness to go along with me.

My concern for Myrna intensified when by the end of two weeks there was no improvement. I increased her drugs to the point of toxicity. She stumbled as she walked with a stiff, masklike face. I ordered other drugs to counter some of the toxic effects of the psychotropic drugs. By the twenty-third day it appeared that electroshock would be necessary. Her eyes had become sunken as she lost more weight. Her tube feedings continued.

When I entered the ward on the twenty-sixth day, I was met with a surprising shout from the nurses.

"Dr. Sherwood," Mrs. Roe said. "Myrna asked for you this morning. She said she had something to tell you. We tried to get her to talk more but she clammed up."

I saw Myrna approaching. Without a word she accompanied me to the interview room. She remained silent for a few moments. She looked puzzled rather than fearful. "Tell me, Dr. Sherwood," she said. "Can I really see my mother? I've been in the hospital nearly four weeks. You said I could go home when I felt better."

She had been lucid throughout her illness, without the disorientation I saw in patients with toxic or organic psychoses. This type of confusion was not part of the acute paranoid schizophrenic reaction that Myrna had been undergoing. Like most schizophrenics, she gave free rein to her wishful fantasies and misinterpreted reality according to her emotional state. Yet she remained fully oriented in all spheres and maintained a modicum of practical common sense. She lived a double psychic existence. This mechanism was an exaggeration of the normal person's use of distortions of reality to suit his needs under emotionally stressful conditions, except that the normal person remains aware of the boundaries of reality.

I now realized that there had been some subtle changes in her affect and thinking over the past few days that had escaped my notice on our daily visits.

"Your mother will be pleased to hear you say you feel better."

"Do you really think she is alive?"

I waited deliberately, not responding to her inquiry. Failure to be positive in my replies would be an error. Yet I wanted Myrna to think again about my daily repeated interpretations of the meaning of her delusional system, the system that appeared to be succumbing to a total and consistent milieu and a dynamic therapeutic approach.

"What makes you feel otherwise, Myrna?" I said. "Please tell me all your feelings." This was my repeated request.

"I'm not sure," she began slowly. "I saw her die, I thought, just before I came in here. She was killed, somehow. I can't remember clearly, but I think I saw it."

"Yes."

"It was like a dream." She paused.

"Yes, a dream, yet it felt very real," I said. "Go on."

"She was attacked—" Again she hesitated. "It's so hard to remember. There was a big man, I think, who crushed her skull with something heavy—a hammer maybe. Yes—that's it—he hit her with a hammer and kept crushing her skull. She screamed, 'My head—it aches so terribly,' and he kept pounding her and pounding her till her head was bloody and her brain—it was like jelly—poured out. It was horrible!" Myrna suddenly began to weep.

"Like a bad dream, yet distant and vague," I said.

"He was a huge man, a giant. I felt so tiny and I was so frightened. I opened my mouth to scream but no sound came out. I tried to run but my legs were stuck. I tried to go for help. But I couldn't move—I couldn't."

"You wanted to help your mother; yet something kept you from it.

Some part of you did not want to help her; a part of you was angry at her."

"It was like a dream," she said, "like a dream and yet I'm not sure it isn't true." She looked at me. She began to breathe harder. Anxiety again began to appear in her eyes.

"Who would want to kill your mother? Who?" Then I saw that I had pushed my patient to deal with her unconscious as hard as I felt she should at one sitting, perhaps too hard. I felt her suspicions rise again. I backed off.

Rarely, with other patients, I had tried to enter the delusional system by agreeing with it to see if the patient would accept me as an ally in that system. By being accepted I might gain access to more of the patient's private thoughts. But this was a potentially dangerous maneuver, for it could reinforce the patient's delusional system and make its ultimate eradication more difficult. With Myrna, my approach had been to attack her delusions while trying to understand them, to allay her anxiety, and to protect her by the reassuring safety of the hospital environment as long as threatening events plagued her. Slowly her fragmented ego began to reconstitute itself. My control of the external world was through hospitalization. My influence on her inner world was through interpretation of her misbeliefs.

"I don't know," she said after a long pause. "I don't know what's true and what isn't."

"We've had enough for now. It's time for lunch," I said, as matter-of-factly as I could.

Myrna left the examining room hesitantly. Instead of returning to her bedroom as she always had following our daily sessions, she walked to the small dining hall. I followed her. The nurses and other patients stopped to look at her. She sat down, picked up a slice of bread, examined both sides, bit off a piece, and slowly chewed it.

"Cheers for Myrna," a male patient sitting at the head of her table said, lifting his orange juice.

"Cheers," a few others replied. Myrna, her face expressionless, lifted her eyes to look at him, but said nothing.

As I entered her room the next morning, Myrna was standing before a mirror, gazing intently at her face as if trying to remember a stranger she had once known. Then she began to comb her light hair, which had hung in disorderly strands.

I decreased her drug dosage before our session began. Now I would probe more intensively. "What else do you remember of your thoughts?" I asked her. "It's important that we understand everything possible about your illness."

She began cautiously. "The giant, he had a horrible leer on his face. He had been planning to kill Mother for some time, I felt. Nothing I could do would stop him."

"Nor did all of you really wish to," I reminded her. "The terrible pounding your mother received on her head was like the terrible headaches she complained of for years, the headaches which began when you were a child." I saw Myrna listening. "But whose face did the giant have? Did you see it?"

"I saw it, but I couldn't tell—for sure—and yet it was a face I knew. He had such a terrible, hateful expression." Myrna's lips parted crookedly. Her white teeth looked fanglike.

"Try to remember," I urged. "Whose face was it?"

"I don't know. It isn't clear, but I'm sure I know him."

"Was it your father's face?"

"No, it couldn't be my father!" She replied quickly, frightened. "He was a giant; my father isn't big. But his expression—maybe— maybe—it was like my father's when he's angry—at her. On no! It couldn't be my father."

"And yet the headaches your mother has come on because of her feelings toward your father which she's afraid to express as anger. You've heard her say, 'My headaches are killing me. My brain is being pounded.' That's the way she described her worst headaches to me."

"Oh no—no—it couldn't be my father!"

"Myrna," I said. "Your unconscious told you what you have denied to yourself—that he might like to see your mother dead. Their marriage has been a bad one. You have reached into your father's unconscious and expressed his secret wish that if she were gone it would solve his problem, too, by relieving him of the guilt of leaving her and the shame of a divorce. And when your own ambivalent wish to destroy your mother arose, your unconscious chose the logical person to be the executioner—your father. You made him a giant to disguise him. And perhaps to your mother he has always been an unconquerable giant. So you began to feel that strangers on the ward, people other than yourself, had 'killed' your mother. Never you."

Myrna stared at me.

"But these are only wishes that you had, Myrna. Wishes that are acceptable because they do not kill, nor come true. Only your own unconscious condemns you. That's why you felt you were going to die. You felt others were going to poison you because you felt responsible for your mother's dreamed-of death. In your delusion you felt that you should be killed for it. But you couldn't allow yourself to connect your fear for your own death with your guilty feelings for her murder. Yet inspite of this, all of your life you have dreaded that she would die."

Myrna still stared. After a while she whispered, "I was always so scared of losing mother."

She continued to confirm my major thesis regarding her delusional withdrawal, beginning with the actual episode of her attempted murder and suicide. We went over other possible events contributory to her illness.

"But it really wasn't me?" she asked, requesting reassurance. "Only part of me wanted to do it? But even that's horrible!"

"Only part of you wanted to destroy your mother because you were so outraged at her, Myrna. No one can condemn your feelings. You will never lose your mother to your nephew or anyone else. Never. Your mother loves you. But you and she need to learn to let go of each other." Myrna nodded. Then she smiled for the first time.

I felt a sense of elation and deep relief as I spoke with her. Myrna sensed it. I suddenly knew we were much closer to each other. My words reached out to touch her. She felt them without retreating. She unconsciously communicated to me that she trusted me and that she recognized that I cared about her.

My terrible fears that she might remain in her psychotic dreamlike world were alleviated.

In the weeks following Myrna's recovery from her delusions, I continued to probe deeply into their meaning, despite her sometimes painful reactions at recollection. If my therapeutic inquiry caused her to suffer a relapse, it was best to have it occur while she was still hospitalized, when I could test how much uncovering was possible.

My work with schizophrenic patients had taught me that the disease was not a distinct entity, but a name applied to people with apparently similar symptoms. The underlying psychopathology was variable, with each patient's illness having a separate and individual etiology. The patient's lifelong family interaction and his constitutional matrix provided the two basic variables in the essentially emotionally determined schizophrenic reaction.

At the end of the third month of Myrna's hospitalization, shortly before she was to leave for home, I discovered another important component of the etiology of her illness.

"I never liked to be away from my mother," Myrna said thoughtfully. "I used to sit and worry about her for hours even when I was little. I can remember how much I wondered what would happen to me if she died. I would be all alone. My father and my little brother—they're like strangers to me. I never got to know either of them."

"You were also scared to leave home for very long?" I asked.

"It still frightens me to be away. When I got out of high school, my father made me go to Bryn Mawr, a fancy women's college in the East. He insisted that I try. My mother knew how I felt and didn't want me to go. She said that I could still live at home and go to a local private college if I wanted to.

"I was miserable and frightened the whole time I was in college. I had dreadful nightmares of people being murdered, even my classmates—almost like," she said slowly, remembering, "almost like what I thought really happened when I came in here. My dreams were always of violence except—except with one of my roommates." She stopped.

"Your dreams about her were different?"

"Yes."

"You felt closer to her?"

Her face flushed. "Not really closer. There were just different kinds of dreams about her."

"Then you had very personal dreams about her?"

Myrna nodded again. "They were only dreams, just dreams of my roommate," she said quickly.

"Caring for you, like your mother?"

"Yes."

"And even being warm to you?"

"Maybe," Myrna said.

"Caressing you and kissing you?"

"How did you know?"

"You said you missed your mother. In your dreams, your roommate became your mother."

"Even kissing me—oh no, it's terrible. I can't talk about it." She shuddered. Then she began to cry softly.

"She was like your mother again, taking care of you."

"Yes," she said, wiping her thin face. "And even more. I even wanted my roommate—I was with her for a year—to kiss me on the lips, my mother never did, and—and down there—and I dreamed of it—all the time—her—some woman—even my mother—kissing me and me kissing her on her private parts—it's too dreadful. I feel so ashamed—I feel—" Her mouth remained open.

"It's your need to be close to a person which you couldn't permit yourself consciously," I said, "to be loved and to be very close to someone. Because of your family's emotional makeup, you developed feelings toward a woman." This part of Myrna's unconscious, like her hostile impulses, needed to be examined so it could become more tolerable to her. I made my acceptance of her repressed homosexual impulses explicit.

"And yet, I never really felt close to my roommate or even to my mother. I can't feel love for anyone, not even my mother. I can't feel any real closeness at all."

"Just a feeling you want to be near your mother."

Her tears arose again. "Only a terrible fear of being alone and my mother being gone! Once when I was just a little girl, maybe nine or ten, I asked my father for a small white kitten because I knew my mother loved our cats. It would be my kitten, my very own. I cuddled it and held it on my lap—the way I saw my mother do. I tried to feel affection for it, but nothing—no feeling—ever came for the kitten— or anyone else. I just pushed it out of my lap. I couldn't feel for anyone. And I can't now either." She covered her face with a wet handkerchief.

Myrna was improving. We had broken the grip of her psychosis. What had done it? Her feeling safe in the hospital and under medical care? The medication? The hospital personnel's and my acceptance of her in spite of her impulses? Some of the observations and comments spoken to Myrna which made her more comfortable and more accepting of herself? Her own recuperative powers? Or a combination of some or all of these factors?

Again I felt the same surge of elation that I sometimes had during my days in general practice when a patient seriously ill, even near death, suddenly took a turn toward recovery.

My flush of enthusiasm propelled me to work harder with her. I now had reason to believe she had a chance for full recuperation, though the delusional system, that strange malady into which some people fall like a mysterious medieval plague, might recur under stress just as unpredictably as it had disappeared. I needed to know more, to pin down more details of her life, past and present, to work with her more intensively, to give her a greater and more authoritative grasp of her illness and its causes and a more profound understanding of her very existence. This would both fortify her recovery and help ward off a recurrence. I worked with Myrna every day, urging her to probe and dig as we searched repeatedly for more pieces of the puzzle.

Again, I questioned her parents. Mrs. McFadden was emotionally drained, a barren desert capable of yielding little more. She merely repeated what she had told me before each time I approached her for information. I finally learned from Mr. McFadden that she and he both had been concealing from me some significant details.

Mr. McFadden and I were alone. "I guess you should know this. I think it's important. My wife was an attractive girl when she was young, but there wasn't much more to her. The truth is, Doctor, Mrs. McFadden became pregnant before we were married.

"We had known each other just a few months. When she discovered she was going to have a baby she became hysterical. She said she'd kill herself because her mother wouldn't live through it. I went into a sweating panic. I knew my father would go into a rage and disinherit me. I had trouble talking with him just as Myrna does with me. I guess it's passed on in the family," he said, looking up. His facial muscles tightened. "I felt sorry for Mrs. McFadden. We were desperate. We decided to get rid of the baby ourselves. What a horrible mistake! She took quinine, castor oil, and every drug we could buy for abortion and nothing did it. This went on for days. All the while she cried and wanted to die. I made her promise not to tell anyone. And one night I finally tried injecting a solution of saline and strong soap into her womb, something a fraternity brother once told me about. Why I tried it myself instead of going to a doctor I'll never know.

"She lay on the floor in the toilet. I had an old medical book to look at. I felt strange, like an abortionist without credentials. I injected the stuff with a big rubber syringe. After a few minutes she cried out with a terrible sudden pain in her chest, and she coughed and said she couldn't breathe. She turned white and I thought she would die right then and there. And then she blacked out.

"I piled her into my car and took her to the nearest doctor, who rushed her to a hospital, where they gave her oxygen and artificial respiration and treated her for shock. That night she nearly died again. The doctors said it was a miracle that she lived. The stuff I injected went into her bloodstream and caused an embolus—I'll never forget that word. You know what that is, don't you?" His face grew even more grave. He stopped speaking.

"Yes, I do," I said.

A collection of the fluid had entered the large, dilated veins of her pregnant uterus and was carried to her lungs, clogging a large blood vessel. Emboli often caused shock, fluid in the lung, necrosis of lung tissue, and sudden death.

"And when it was over, she was still pregnant. It was a miracle she was alive. I decided I had to marry her. I was frightened about the whole thing—her nearly dying, and of the police, and of her parents pressing charges. It was all hushed up when I married her. My family paid the police off. They agreed to keep it quiet and her parents, though troubled, were pacified by the marriage.

"She said she loved me, but my family never forgave her. They blamed her, not me. 'She trapped you—that cheap prostitute,' my mother said. My family had a name and they expected me to marry someone of social class. Mrs. McFadden's father operated a metal lathe on the assembly line at Douglas. I wasn't ready to settle down. I really hated the marriage and the baby, but Mrs. McFadden insisted she loved me and said I'd learn to love her, too. I never did. And that's where Myrna comes in. Poor kid lost out right from the start with two miserable parents.

"I know my wife cried and carried on when I went out with other women, but she said she didn't want a divorce. She always hoped it would work out, and with a baby and all, and with her family being poor, I guess she had little choice. She kept insisting I'd learn to love her.

"She worried about our marriage constantly and cried and looked blue all the time and never paid much attention to the child. Or she'd suddenly grab the baby and smother her, and love her up, and sleep with her and wouldn't let her go—telling a two-month-old baby about her own sorrows."

Tears came to his eyes. He choked. "The worst began one night after I'd had a few drinks. I was sick of the marriage. Myrna was only about three or four months old. I told Mrs. McFadden that I wished she had died during the abortion, that I felt like killing her now anyway, that I never did love her and never could. I told her that my family thought she was a harlot. Mrs. McFadden turned away from me and collapsed in her chair without a word. She actually fainted. I've seen her faint several times since then. I was very angry at her. I resented the whole thing right from the start, and I told her what was in my guts, that I married her out of guilt and pity."

A hoarse sob escaped from his throat. He caught himself and stopped. "I never paid any attention to the baby. I abhorred her—a little baby." His voice broke again. "And the poor kid had done nothing except to be born."

He had a need to tell all. I became aware of his enormous grief. A tight sensation arose in my chest.

"I never paid much attention to her as a baby, or as a little kid either—only when she became older. And from the day I told Mrs. McFadden I hated her, she just shriveled up inside herself—and her headaches began. And as for Myrna—she just seemed to stare at the baby for weeks and weeks after that—never picked her up anymore. I became sorry about what I said, even if it was the truth.

"Mrs. McFadden just sat in one chair all day long and Myrna began to cry a lot and vomit and refuse food, and though Mrs. McFadden didn't say anything to anyone about our quarrel, I felt her withdraw from the baby more and more as if she had no feeling for the child or anything else.

"If Myrna cried, she had the housekeeper feed her or she made a half-assed attempt to feed her herself—but nothing more—no playing or pleasure in the baby—just as if the baby were only an object that needed winding. Then sometimes she would grab Myrna fitfully and love her up again for a while and cry pitifully with the child in her arms, and then she'd push the child away. Myrna's feeding and sleeping grew worse by the day. She whined and fretted all the time. The pediatrician couldn't find anything wrong. I could see what was going on, but I was sick of the whole thing and I just stayed away from home as much as I could, and Mrs. McFadden became a zombie stoned by drugs for years.

"I always had a girl friend, but along came Leslie a few years later—probably when I was drinking too much again one night. It's been a strange marriage. With the kids there, something just wouldn't let me get a divorce, and as the years went by, my children began to mean more to me—"

The tears rolled down his face. "I hope it's not too late for Myrna. I've never been much of a father to her."

Now it was clear. The terrible closeness to her mother was not love but a dread of detachment from the one object in her life that had any meaning for her. The earliest type of relationship between mother and infant—a symbiosis, with mother or mother substitute and child enjoying a mutual feeling of closeness—had in Myrna's case become pathological. Under healthy circumstances during the symbiotic phase the helpless infant is dependent on its mother for indispensable nurturing, protection, and love, and the mother is "dependent" on the infant for a nearly equally indispensable return supply of warmth and joy. Around the end of the first year this symbiosis lessens and the infant separates from its mother to explore the world, returning to her only when it becomes fearful or needful. Part of Myrna had never grown beyond the symbiotic phase because Myrna's mother had caused her infant daughter to be continually overwhelmed with anxiety.

Her mother's agitated and depressed preoccupation with her marital life and her inconsistent dealing with Myrna resulted in Myrna's remaining in a state of perpetual anxiety during the critical developmental years of infancy and early childhood. This anxiety prevented Myrna from experiencing and integrating the customary events of childhood under even remotely optimal conditions. Instead, Myrna had erected an unusual superstructure of adaptive defenses, which forced her to cope with life in a crippled fashion. Her ego, which was responsible for the executive functioning of her personality, was weak, fragmentary, and poorly developed and organized. At a moment of great personal stress, the whole structure came tumbling down in one disintegrating crash. In her psychotic state, she was unable to distinguish reality from the fantasies of her imagination, much as a normal person is unable to do while dreaming. Some of her psychic growth had been arrested or distorted at the earliest stages, even before the development of formal language; these defects revealed themselves in her psychotic confusion with its frequently personal symbolic content.

Myrna's mother unconsciously had tied Myrna to her with a bond of fearful dependency and secondarily wished for homosexual gratification as a replacement for maternal security and love. Her mother's emotional avarice was a reaction to her own limited need-fulfillment from a poor marital relationship. It was also a residue of problems from her youth which she had hoped to overcome through marriage. Myrna had inherited the difficulties of her parents' past.

Unfortunately, her father had been incapable of acting as a need-satisfying replacement for mother. Nor did Myrna learn to love him as a girl must learn to love her father before she can feel for another man. Her parents' preoccupation with their own difficulties left little room for sensitivity to the emotional needs of their first-born child.

The second child, born under a different familial circumstance, largely escaped the destructive stresses of his sister's early life.

During the weeks before she left the hospital, both parents visited frequently and Myrna went home on short day visits. She maintained her recovery, and I was willing to risk discharging her about three months after her admission.

The day of her discharge, Myrna waved to me as she waited for the nurse to unlock the door of the corridor of the hospital; a slight yet spontaneous smile was on her lips. Her face no longer bore the sad and serious gaze which had been hers for so long. "I'll be there Tuesday," she reminded me, "at your office." We were to continue her treatment, including intensive psychotherapy; she knew we were still at the beginning.

I waved back to her and said, "See you then, Myrna." I was aware that her struggle would take a long time, and that we, Myrna and I, had much of her past to relive, her present to reshape, and her future to redirect.

Chapter 12
Faith the Man-Eater

She shifted in her chair. Her green-blue eyes and black hair were set on a symmetrical oval face with perfect features. Her figure, carriage, and vivacity were those of a college coed. Only the lines around her eyes and on her forehead betrayed her to be a woman in her mid-forties. She smoked slowly, one cigarette after another, as she spoke facing me.

"It's what went on one afternoon in a restaurant that brings me in to see you, Doctor. John—my best friend's husband—and I were alone. He's a physician, of sorts."

"How long have we known each other, Faith?" John said to me, finishing his salad.

"It must be twenty years at least," I said, munching mine. "Don't you remember—just a month before you and Louise were married?"

"Yes, now I remember," he said in a low voice. "Louise had spoken of you so many times before. She said she was afraid to introduce you to me because she didn't want to let me see how beautiful you were. 'My roommate looks like Scarlet O'Hara in *Gone with the Wind*,' she would say.

"But Faith," he suddenly pleaded, "why shouldn't we? You're not in love with Fred. I know you aren't. I've been watching you these last few years."

"This certainly hasn't been a romantic proposition on your part," I said. I couldn't keep from smiling. "I doubt if any other woman has ever tried to digest such a spicy proposal from the husband of her closest friend along with her salad and mayonnaise in the middle of Scandia in broad daylight while they were waiting for their respective husband and wife. This could bring on abdominal cramps, couldn't it, Doctor John?"

Faith laughed confidently in the manner of a woman who is aware that men still stare at her.

"But," I smiled, "of all people, for you, an obstetrician, to make a pass! You've seen more nude women than a masseuse at La Paz—what makes you still sexually curious? Why would you want to go to bed with me? You can have your pick of the pelvics you do—isn't that what you call it when you put a woman on the examining table and stab her with your clammy fingers?"

"Faith, don't tease me," he said. "Please. You know how carefully I've managed to have the four of us meet somewhere, once or twice a week for years now, and—"

"Yes, I know," I said. "And I think Louise knows too, somewhere inside of her. Yet she continues as if she didn't. Any woman can sense it if she allows herself to. Strange, she and I have had so much in common since we met at Radcliffe. We lived together in a dorm for four years, and walked side by side on graduation day. Then we both came back to Southern California, and each of us married a man destined to become successful and wealthy, and settled down to luxurious and pretentious lives in Beverly Hills. And now, one of these men wants to make it with both of us—though, I assume, one at a time."

"But if you do care for me why shouldn't we have a relationship—a relationship of two mature adults who are attracted to one another?"

"So all you want is a grown-up, mature 'relationship'—take me to bed like a college boy of twenty-one, you purveyor of the Pill, but we won't call it an 'affair.' Sophisticated people have better words for it. You say you love me, but 'no complications—marriages and children and divorces are all so complex.' Haven't we talked enough of this, my dear Doctor John? Shouldn't we abort the subject?"

"Faith, please. You're always laughing at me. I really do love you. But don't you see, I'm fifty-four, and six months from now I'll be a grandfather. It's hard to think of starting all over again in a marriage—even with a woman ten years younger."

"Yet, it might be interesting to go to bed with you. I've never been to bed with a grandfather before!" She smiled musingly. "Imagine, your daughter Rosalie having a baby! I've had a hand in helping you and Louise bring her up, and now she's twenty and married and about to make me a 'great aunt.' And her father wants to make me too—like one man's family. It's all so rapturously incestuous and deliciously exciting. I assume, with all the energy so much planning requires, that you must be very fiery in bed. The man with the cold steel speculum becomes hot."

"But if you're so unhappy," John asked, "why do you stay with Fred?"

"I didn't know it showed so much," I said. I felt my anger rise. "Your proposition is hardly a flattering one. You ask to have an affair with no commitments—you're used to affairs. It doesn't mean much more to you than putting another female on your table and doing your sleight-of-hand. You may see a lot of women undressed, but we're not really naked. You can't see much of us that way. Sometimes, though, we pretend so that we don't even see ourselves. Take Louise, married twenty-one years to you, friends twenty-five years with me, and she even arranges to provide us with the symbolic shovel to dig her marital grave." I held up a spoon. "'Whoever meets first go ahead and eat,' Louise said to me on the phone last night. 'I may be a little late for lunch tomorrow.'"

"Faith, you really do have a cruel streak in you," he said. "You taunt me, even though you know how much I really care."

"Being accused of cruelty by a dull physician who can speak only in clichés, even while he tries to proposition you, is both tedious and annoying. I'm not sure you could do much in bed anyway," I said. "So many men grow limp after forty, I hear. My poor, poor Fred. He tries but he can't quite make it. I suspect you might have the same problem. Maybe that's why men like you are always looking for other women." He ignored my words, but I know that I got to him. I could see it on his face.

"But why did you marry him?" he said. "I had the feeling you never really did love him, even when I first knew you. You had your choice of almost any man you wanted. I know Fred couldn't help but be a successful attorney. He simply joined his father's law firm. Was it just his wealth? Why did you marry him?"

I waited a long while before answering. "For an obstetrician on the make with his wife's best friend you are a most curious curiosity. Maybe success and comfort did mean a lot to me. I never cared to struggle, you know. Scarlet O'Hara never did either. But you, my dear handsome doctor, why did you marry a simple little college girl destined to become a third-grade teacher?"

"Simple," he repeated, taken by my description. "Yes, I suppose that's the way most people see Louise—simple."

"Yes, uncomplicated, sweet, and even mildly attractive. She's never been and never will be competition for me or any other woman. That's what drew me to her most. I knew she would always be a loyal friend. As you see, I'm partial to loyalty. It's that and her simplicity that I think I like best in her. Tell me, why did you marry her?"

"I suppose," he said thoughtfully, "part of it is the lonely, desperate life of the medical student, a hermit year after year, no time to date or see women unless your cadaver happens to be female. And I suppose her childlike quality attracted me too. I cherished that in her—then."

"And now you're bored, aren't you? Now the successful and much sought-after obstetrician, the chief-of-staff of Longview Hospital, a clinical professor at the university, is wealthy, busy, and bored. I'm not sure it's really I whom you seek, anyway. I may only be a character in the beautiful and luxurious daydream of a life, the life that you as a hungry, poor medical student envied, and that you still pursue, even though you have it now."

"Tell me, Faith, if we had it to do all over again, and you knew what I would become someday, would you have married me?"

"You mean if I had known how numbing it would be to be the wife of a successful attorney for twenty years, would I have traded all of those rich, luxurious, boring years for years of struggle with a young medical student—living in a tiny, dim-lit apartment wearing old worn-out dresses, my face a sweet, sweating mess, listening to the neighbors quarreling and their children screeching and crying, and smelling Mrs. McQuain's cabbage soup from down the hallway, and doing the cleaning and washing, and ironing your three shirts every week for school?"

"You know, Faith, your frankness touches me, as it always has—so fierce and so forthright."

At that moment Louise entered and saw us. Fred followed a moment later. Louise said, "You two been waiting long? You seem to have been engaged in some serious conversation. I saw you as I came in."

"No," said I. "Only the usual trivia that a married woman discusses with a married man while they wait for their wife and husband to join them."

"So you see, Doctor, even my best friend's husband craves me. He says he loves me and wants an affair, but I'm hardly attracted to him.

And yet I have him trapped, same as I do nearly every man with whom I want to play. Neither John, nor Louise, nor my husband suspect that I've had dozens of affairs since I've been married, and that's why I'm here. You and I, Doctor, need to understand why I'm compelled to entice men into bed with me, even when I find most of them to be simpering and asinine."

Faith's candor and directness were appealing. These qualities, combined with her wit and beauty, made me understand how easily men would be drawn to her until they felt her sting.

This was our second meeting.

"Since the beginning of my marriage I've been in control," she said. "Fred always waited on me and worshiped me. I knew that this was the kind of man I would have to marry."

"You mean," I said, "his wealth was not the only reason you married him?"

"Yes, there was more to it. I was attracted to a few men when I was younger, many of them wealthy, most of them more appealing than Fred. But I didn't want to marry any of them. Once I was married their propositions didn't stop either, much to my surprise. I've been asked to bed by men who I never dreamed did such things. I'm used to it now. Despite their marital facade, they all seem to be on the make. But I'm a good one to scoff at them." She laughed. "Innocent me."

"Your cynicism applies to all men?"

"Of course it does. I simply do what men do, tit for tat." A quick smile crossed her face again.

"Hmm! How do you manage to avoid being caught by your husband?"

"He doesn't indicate that he's aware. Not in the slightest. He never questions where I've been or what I've done, even when I come home at three o'clock in the morning. 'Out with the girls,' is what I tell him, and that's all there is to it. Fred is just plain Fred, dull but always there. He would do anything for me, and most people think him a very capable attorney, even though he inherited his father's law firm. What more could a woman want?"

"And you say you've never wanted children?"

"No, though I've been pregnant twice."

"Two pregnancies, lost?"

"No, almost found." She laughed again. "Fred didn't even know I was pregnant. Both times I obtained abortions, not secretive

Mexican or back-alley abortions, but the very best Beverly Hills had to offer, with the top gynecologists, long before abortions were legal, and John, mind you, was not among the doctors who did them."

I found myself observing her intently. She enjoyed performing, gripping me with the same suave mastery she claimed to have over other men, though I gave no sign that I was either startled or amused. That would only feed her exhibitionism. I was deeply curious as to what motivated her unusual sexual behavior and her husband's blindness. Was there a *folie à deux* which permitted her acting out? Did he unconsciously approve of her actions, even promote them?

"Why didn't you tell Fred of your abortions?" I asked.

"Because he wasn't the father," she replied.

At our next meeting Faith said, "You'd be surprised, Doctor, at some of the men I've gone out with, some of the most respectable names in town. I had a serious affair with one of the chief executives at McDonnell-Douglas. And there have even been a few medical doctors on my list, including one psychiatrist."

She looked at me accusingly, but with a touch of triumph in her voice. "It was years ago. I went for therapy before, you see. My first psychiatrist was a psychoanalyst like you, but stuffy; he made all the classical interpretations that I had read in Freud. The next one was more interesting, but I had a disagreement with him. He demanded that I stop seeing Bill, the executive. Psychiatrists shouldn't tell patients what to do, should they?" She waited.

I said nothing.

"No reply, Doctor?" she persisted.

"You always want to make certain," I said, "that you are in control of every situation, even at this moment, so all decisions involving you will be yours no matter how many others are affected. But what if I disagree with you? Does that mean you'll run from therapy again?"

"Perhaps not, if you make sense," she answered, shrugging impatiently.

She had expressed a desire to explore her problems, but her intense hostility made me equally aware of her readiness to quit. I felt myself growing irritated at her; why was she taking up my time, interesting as she may be, when she was so likely to flee therapy once we had begun? Did she simply wish to test me before she could trust me? Or was her major purpose to control me and to play with me and with therapy? Why had she come to see me anyway? I was just another psychiatrist.

I knew I had to be careful to avoid antagonizing her, at least initially, to keep from giving her the impetus to abandon therapy for good. Maybe that was it? She wished to convince herself once and for all that she had given psychotherapy a fair trial and that psychiatry had failed, not she. I knew from her incomplete history that her anger might become intense if I made premature interpretations which displeased her. I had to be certain that our relationship was strong enough to bind her to the treatment. I had to seek out and carefully nurture that part of her which was dissatisfied with her own behavior.

"My third psychiatrist, the last one I had, he and I worked for over half a year. After a few months he said that he had become fascinated by me, that I was the most interesting woman he had ever treated. He warned me from the onset that his treatment was unorthodox, that he varied it according to his patient's requirement. We began to have sexual relations right in his office. He said it was to teach me how to feel about men, to learn what it was to love and to relate rather than to just 'act out,' and that I would be a better wife for it, ultimately. He was a psychiatrist, highly qualified, I thought. He had a wife, but she was not very warm, he said. He stayed married for the sake of their children, whom he loved. After a good while of his therapy, I decided that I wouldn't be seeing him any longer and that my 'treatment' was over and so was his. He agreed to stopping my therapy, but he wanted to continue seeing me."

She paused, watching for my reaction.

"You stopped seeing him?"

"Yes. I decided that he wasn't ethical. Sounds contradictory, my having an affair with my psychiatrist, then telling him he wasn't ethical. During my therapy, I thought he was amusing. Then I realized that my original reason for seeing him was being defeated and I grew angry. Are there many psychiatrists who have affairs with their patients, Doctor?"

"How did you come to see this doctor?" I asked, without answering. "Were you referred to him by someone?"

"No, I discovered him, or should I say uncovered him, on my own. I thought I would try someone I chose, this time. I didn't ask my own physician a third time. I dislike being referred to someone as if I were some chattel to be sent here and there at some other man's whim. And yet I decided I should work with a psychiatrist. I'm here because Louise once heard John mention you. Neither of them knows I'm here, though."

"But why did you choose to begin with your last psychiatrist?"

She hesitated. "He—he seemed more interesting—less doctrinaire. I had no idea what would—"

"More interesting because you sensed he would fall prey to you," I added. "So you defeated him and your therapy. Maybe you weren't deeply interested in therapy at that time anyway. Without being fully aware, part of you was primarily bent on defeating your psychiatrist, the way you've defeated so many other men, humiliating them and proving them inadequate."

Her history, though unusual, was believable. I was struck by how she told her tale: with the flamboyance of a thirteen-year-old girl whom I had once seen together with her parents. The girl confessed to me how she deliberately burned her home to the ground, turning to scrutinize her parents' faces to enjoy their horror.

I wondered if I'd gone too far so early in our work. No. I decided I hadn't. She said she desired to stop her sexual conquests, but her history and attitude said otherwise. I expected that soon she would have contempt for me, too, either by her attempted sexual conquest and abandonment of me, or by her finding me dull or disagreeable. I also wondered about the sources of her strong compulsion to destroy men. She had already searched for and found the rare psychiatrist whom she could ensnare and then deem culpable despite her collusion in his actions.

She glanced at me harshly, then recovered and gathered up her charm. "Yes, I have been critical of men. But they generally were deserving of it. So you think I'm out to defeat them, do you? That's a unique thought. I'll look into it." She stared at me.

At this moment, I felt the iciness inside her that lived alongside her charm and wit. The bit of warmth that I had felt in her a moment ago had disappeared.

She began our next session by replying to my inquiry about her husband. "What more do you want to know about him? He has a kind of understanding combined with obtuseness that tends to suit me very well. I've known some men who tell their wives what friends to have, what to do during the day, when and if they can have a new car or even go to the bathroom. I couldn't stand that. I've been my own person since I was a child and I don't intend to change. Fred knows I enjoy myself at a hotel occasionally at the cocktail hour with whomever I please and this isn't going to change. Fred's only objection, when I've gotten home, is my having had a cocktail or two more than I should, but that's no real problem."

"What do you mean 'no real problem'?"

"I've been stopped by some zealous policemen once or twice for drunk driving, but Fred took care of that. And once I drove a little fast going home from a man's apartment. It was late at night and rounding a curve, my white Cadillac—I loved that car—spun out into a ditch, turned over a few times and was flattened out. I wasn't hurt, but the car was a total wreck. That frightened me. I take no more than just a few drinks now, usually, except when I forget, or I'm angry at someone. Fred is what a husband should be and there isn't much more to be said about him."

"What work does he do?"

"His firm specializes in corporate law—such complicated matters. He and my father talk about this for hours when my parents come in from Chicago. My father and Fred have some business interests in common but nothing more. It's hard to see how my mother could have been married to a man like my father for forty-five years! He's such an unbearable person. He still keeps her on a tight budget to run their home. Every check has to be listed in a ledger. If she overspends by five dollars a week, his face grows red and he huffs and puffs and screams and pounds. The housekeeper and my mother hide in terror in one of the back bedrooms till he's finished. He wants to know where every dollar goes, and why the hell she fails to plan, and why she needs a new coat when she just bought a mink three years ago. And on and on.

"My mother has never been able to stand up to him. She creeps around on tiptoe to please him. Yet she says she's always gotten all the things she wants, but in her own way and in her own time. That's not for me, being a cautious cat in fear of the house dog." Now Faith laughed. "Even though she really is a sly kitten. You see, my father is in the auto parts business. Their lives revolved around auto parts." Her cheeks flushed red, anger accentuating her green-blue eyes.

"When I was twelve I swore my life would be different. They love each other, my mother's always said, but I've wondered. His ancestry is Scotch-English. She dances to his bagpipes like a fallen woman because her grandfather was a lowly Frenchman and her father was poor. She shushes me up when I tell her that, but it's true. They've always had more than enough, but since they were married, he hoards his money in secret places unknown to her. The only reason they had me is because my mother begged him for a child. So he satisfied her. He would have been content to live alone with her and a house full of shock absorbers. If I had been a newly designed auto muffler he would've paid more attention to me.

"He felt kids should be neither seen nor heard nor smelt, even babies. He thought I never made sense, and that children were meddlesome, distasteful little things. I remember his teasing me now and then, the only recognition I ever received from him, but largely he lived as if I had never been alive. I never had a meaningful conversation with him in my life. I retreated when he came home from work and I began to hate him from the time I was that big. I think my mother cared for me, but she was such a helpless, poor, soft, dumb little thing, so in awe of him that she couldn't conceive of any independent right of her own in the household. 'Life with Father' wasn't like the play, centering around a lovable, benevolent tyrant. My father was a seclusive, unsmiling monster.

"When I was very little it was constantly, 'Your father's tired,' or 'Don't bother Father; he's busy.' Who the hell wanted to bother him? Bothering him was just to say a word or two, to talk and be heard. In later years it was, 'Let Daddy rest—no friends over now. He's had a hard week. Just the three of us this weekend.' When was it anything but 'the three of us'?: I in my room alone after supper, and the two of them in the library. My mother sensed our antagonism from my youngest years. She quietly tried to keep me in another part of the house. He controlled her completely, and she let him do it, and I hated her for it. He thought he still had me under his cold finger even when I grew older. But I fixed him. I remember how much I loathed him over the years and how I schemed to take over my own life. When I grew into my teens I started to sneak out my bedroom window after they went to bed.

"My bedroom was way down the hall at the end of our house. It was a big, sprawling old home on Lake Michigan. I remember I was fourteen because I'd just started to menstruate, and I had convinced my mother to let me trade my bedroom for the old housekeeper's east room. I said I liked the sunlight coming into my bedroom early in the morning. After they all went to bed, I'd be gone, joy riding with some kids from school, and we'd drink and raise hell till 2:00 A.M. And then I'd sneak back in through the window, put the screen back on, and they would never know the difference. We did that at opportune times at least once or twice a month for years."

"And you never got caught?"

"Not till I was seventeen and then only by a fluke. After I went to bed in my part of the house, I was the forgotten child, gone to the tomb. I'd usually put a couple of pillows under the blankets in case our half-blind old housekeeper, Brigette, or my mother ever came up to see me after bedtime, something they rarely did. Brigette would take a quick look from the doorway, see a lump under the blankets, and tiptoe away." She laughed.

"One night, though, my girl friend's mother called my home at one o'clock in the morning. She woke my mother up and asked if Helen was sleeping over. Helen and I, we raised hell together. Helen would tell her mother she was sleeping over at my house. I'd cover up for her when she wanted to spend the night with her boyfriend. This was in the days when I was finally allowed to have a friend sleep over. That night Helen and I had supper at my house, said good night to my mother, and went to bed. Except we took off in her red Chevy as soon as everyone was asleep. A snoopy old aunt of hers saw Helen's car parked on the wrong side of town with no one around and called Helen's mother, who was getting suspicious anyway. My mother and dad got up, came into my room, lifted the covers up and saw that the lumps were only pillows, and had a series of convulsions.

"When we came back they were waiting outside in the driveway for us with poison in their hearts. My father's face was filled with rage. I didn't have to go through the inconvenience of crawling back through the window that night. My father raced me through the doorway. It was a tie. He caught me and beat me with his fists till I couldn't move; he said I was the village whore and locked me in my room for a week. I wasn't even allowed to go to school. My mother just cried, but as usual, she was afraid to say anything to him and, really, though she didn't like to see her daughter bleeding except from proper places, she was just as vindictive as my father that time."

Faith clenched her fist, her jaw tightened, and her beautiful face was gone. In its place was an asymmetric, muscular grimace. Her voice was low and husky. "I hated him so God-damned much, I can still feel it." A partial smile returned. "I swore to them on my life that I was still a virgin. I wonder if either of them really believed me. My father kept chopping away at me for months, asking if I had ever been out like that before. Again and again I swore I never had been, though my virginity and I both had been gone long before that night.

"All that he cared about was his reputation in the neighborhood, if he cared about anything. Out came all his seventeen years of hatred and resentment for the child who intruded upon his marriage. He always wanted my mother all to himself—I'm sure of it. He ignored me all my life till he started searching for my maidenhead. Why was it that it meant so much to him or anyone else for that matter?

"Isn't a woman creature entitled to the same sexual pleasure as a man creature? I signed the Magna Charta of women's lib before most women knew they were enslaved. And my mother," she pursed her lips, emphasizing every word harshly, "my sweet—dar-ling mo-ther is the Benedictine Arnold of the women's revolution. She's a good little soldier and she serves everything my father wants from his cocktails to his cock, his every whim.

"You're shocked at my language, aren't you? I told you I've despised my father since I was six years old. Whenever a woman friend said anything against men's domination of the world my mother looked up in utter horror. 'Husbands work so terribly hard and we have to do all we can to make their lives easier.' Well, here's one girl who doesn't think so. Husbands don't deserve one bit more than wives. My mother might have been satisfied with her role, but I swore I'd never be and so here I am Doc-tor Sher-wood. Here I am, joint chief-of-staff of women's rights." She laughed and lit a cigarette. "And while you're trying to figure me out, how about giving me an ashtray before my droppings dirty your nice beige carpets."

"I brought my husband here today, as you requested," Faith said. Fred V. Jensen was a slender-faced man of medium height with a short, thin nose, narrow, grey eyes, and a serious disposition. He arose silently, gave a lukewarm, flaccid handshake, entered my consultation room, sat down, and waited expectantly for me to begin. Faith remained in the waiting room beyond his hearing.

"Thank you for coming, Mr. Jensen," I said. "I asked you here to get your view of Mrs. Jensen's problems."

He remained silent for a long while.

"What has she told you, Doctor?" He began in a soft voice, looking away from me except for occasional glances.

I avoided a direct answer. I wanted to probe his view of Faith. "She has some personal feelings that are troubling her. I thought you might be able to help me understand her."

"She does drink a bit too much occasionally. I've talked with her about it more than once."

"How often does it happen?"

"Not too much now. She had a bad accident a few months ago and she cut down some—maybe once a month or so. Other than that I'm not sure why she's here. Oh, we do have a little sex problem, though. Or maybe it really isn't a problem. I've never been highly sexed and I have trouble sometimes. But she never complains about it. That's all I can think of."

"You've never been highly sexed?" I repeated. He was parrying with me. He still tried to ferret out what Faith had told me. I knew that I would learn very little from him by pressing for information. Candor was the most effective way to bring a response if I were to get one.

"I know that this is a difficult area for you. Mrs. Jensen has already gone into it a bit with me—your problem in obtaining an erection. But this is no problem for the two of you, you say?"

"I'm not sure. She never complains. We have sex only once in a while, maybe every few months—even longer sometimes. Did she tell you that she was dissatisfied?"

"No, she said nothing like that. Don't the two of you then have an understanding about sexual matters between you?"

"Yes, I guess we do," he said quietly. "We have enough other interests to satisfy us both: an exceptional home, a yacht, and a broad social life. So I guess we're not as sexual as most people are. I know it's unusual, but we've always had the understanding that you mention, Doctor. I let her know before we married that I wouldn't be like most men, jealous of her independence, or always looking for sex, or trying to keep her locked in the house. That's not my style and she's happy with me. She does spend quite a bit of money on clothing and things like that, but we have means, and we manage all right. I'd say, all in all, we have a good marriage." He stared ahead, then looked at me blandly.

"Then you have no particular complaints about Mrs. Jensen or the relationship you have with her?"

"No, no complaints. Maybe she also wants to straighten out some of her feelings about her mother and dad. Her father's a very strong person. She said she never was able to get along with him, so she looked for the kind of husband who would be unlike him. He hates little children—thinks every human ought to be born a male at least twenty-one years of age, hard-working, and Republican. To this day he thinks she should ask my permission when she goes out of the house—fails to understand how I could allow Faith to go to Spain for a month alone in the summer, but I've explained to him my law firm requires my presence nearly constantly. Once in a while we go together somewhere for the weekend, but she insists that she can go whenever and wherever she wants. I try not to keep her. Faith's mother never approves of Faith going on vacations alone either— quiet little woman, she is. Faith fought with her mother all through her childhood to get her mother to stand up against her father, but she never would.

"During her early years Faith went to a private day school for girls, wore a white-and-green uniform, and hated every hour of it. The neighborhood she lived in had high-fenced yards with guard dogs and locked front gates. Aside from the girls in school she rarely saw other kids except when she was a teenager. Then they let her keep company with one older girl up the hill who was the studious kind. She never got out of the house to date or see other friends till she went off to Radcliffe where I met her. I was a law student at Harvard. We started dating then and continued when we came back to California. We had an agreement that she wouldn't be incarcerated after we were married. She hated that so much in her childhood."

Again he became silent. He sat up stiffly in his thick, dark suit, looking formal and proper like a barrister in a nineteenth-century British novel.

The understanding between them, as Faith had said, was made quite explicit at the onset of their life together. Fred had consented because of his own intrapsychic needs, including, I guessed, his fear of impotence. Faith suited him well. She was in society's view a beautiful wife who accompanied him to social gatherings and business events. In their private life she would not demand that he perform sexually; nor did she ever trouble him to discuss the sexual aspects of their marriage. Faith was totally free to explore and experiment in attempting to satisfy her own emotional needs.

When our meeting ended, Fred left without saying goodbye.

"Why," asked Faith in our next session, "do I want treatment now? That's a good question, Doctor. As you say, I've had what I seemed to want all these years. And why did I see these other doctors and why you now? You say I've defeated all the other doctors so that any treatment would fail?"

"Yes, the other doctors fell prey to you, and I would suspect a part of you wants to destroy me, also, despite your statement that this time you really want to 'work with a psychiatrist,' to work out your problems with men. Look at the important men in your life. Your husband is passive and nondemanding as you told me. He gives you all the freedom you desire, lets you control your marriage, and is content for his own reasons to give you your way in every matter. Your father ignored you or was hostile and resentful toward you. He never really wanted children."

"Same as Fred," she said. "He has no more interest in raising children than in raising rhinoceroses. How did you find Fred?"

"Much as you described him. I wanted to tell you what our meeting was about. We spoke of your family and their relationship with you, and—"

"Fred still looks upon me as being innocent, doesn't he?"

"Yes, he does. I, of course, revealed nothing about you that contradicted this."

"I have no concern about that, Doctor. You say I've never been close to any man, that I've used them, seduced them, then spat upon them?"

"Yes, as many men use women, only this time it was you, a woman, who fucked them. It becomes clearer with your history, you need to reverse the roles and be on top. You want to usurp the traditional role of the man and—"

"You're right. Even in sexual relations the only way I've ever had an orgasm is by being on top. Uh! I don't like their clumsy, heavy bodies weighing me down. I have to feel free."

"To be in control of your pleasure and of theirs," I said. "But sexuality is only one aspect of human relationships and often largely a symbolic one. There may be something even more basic to male-female and all human relationships."

"What do you mean? I thought sexual attitudes were about as basic as things can be between men and women!"

"Yes," I said, "but what preceded your sexual attitudes and what helped to formulate them? Certainly there must be a representative of your early relationship with your father contained within your psyche. This had to do with the earliest attitudes and feelings and even sensations toward him. But even more primitive formulations of your identity as a human being preceded your sexual identity. Your sexual identity, like most people's, and your choice of sexual objects developed in your later infancy and early childhood at ages two, three, four, five, six, and so on. Its structure includes those earliest nonsexual, interpersonal feelings and attitudes, amalgamated with your later experiences, derived from continuing relationships with your father and mother and other men and women.

"For you, men are contemptible, hateful, and untrustworthy. They only use women, as your father demonstrated to you. In your unconscious he is the prototype of all men, though intellectually you know otherwise. You even know other women love men, but you don't believe it. You feel your mother never really loved your father but only exploited him. You feel she is faking it, even though she said she 'loved him in her own way.' You fail to believe she loves him because you could never experience a feeling of love for him yourself—only anger and resentment or indifference. So you developed the unconscious assumption that affection for men existed only in words—spoken or written by poets and deceivers. You told me that you question even Louise's love for John, though you sense it might be real."

"You read me well," she said. "My puzzlement over Louise is one reason I'm here. I've known her for all these years, yet I've doubted her words about her love toward John or her affection for me. Down deep I'm aware she is the most genuine person I've ever known— maybe the only one. I've seen her weep real tears at Rosalie's humiliation when she failed one year in high school and when a boyfriend whom Rosalie loved dropped her, hurting Rosalie deeply. And I've seen her fret about John when she saw him grow weary of his work, not because of what his unhappiness might do to her, but what it might do to him." Faith's words stopped abruptly.

When she started talking again, she appeared to be speaking to herself. "So you think I'm here because I've never really learned to care about a man?" She was silent for another few moments.

"You must wonder why my friendship with Louise has this much meaning for me. I wonder too." She drew a long, thin cigarette from a package in her purse, lit it, took one puff, and crushed it in an ashtray.

"I guess this is why I've really come back to see someone like you; I've become annoyed at myself and tired of my life. As I said, Louise is the only person I've ever really trusted. I've tried her and tested her and she remains loyal. And for the most frivolous reason, an interesting escapade with another man, her husband, I considered betraying her, when I've had all sorts of men chasing me my whole life. I take my pick and play with them, and they play with me, and then I get rid of them, and that's the end. Every time I think I'm beginning the meaningful chapter in my life it runs just a few pages, sometimes only a few paragraphs, and when it's over I try to re-read it and understand it, and it's all just gibberish. Maybe now at the age of forty-two, when I realize that stealing men from other women can last only a few years longer, I want to begin a different sort of life with someone—something with more substance."

"Not with Fred?"

"No, not Fred. It couldn't work. Fred and I were a compromise for each other, a compromise made twenty years ago. I can't see how I could possibly really fall in love with him."

"Fred was an investment you made in earlier days when you wanted insurance for yourself, not a marriage: an investment that paid off well in social advancement and material comfort. So you think you're ready for a change? After twenty years?"

"I'm not sure. There's a sadness in it—for Fred I mean—after this long. He has less chance than I do. I don't know what would happen to him if I left." She waited. "You know, Doctor, you've asked for my fantasies. Here's one: men were always an institution for me. Not people, but creatures. When I saw one I liked, I said to myself, 'Get him.' Getting him means having him become attached to me. If a man I fancied failed to go after me, I'd feel very hurt, but I'd quickly dismiss him from my mind because I knew another would come along soon. No one could hurt me for very long. I'd play a game with myself—a game of how many men were chasing me. If one dropped me, one or two others would pick up the chase so that there was always somebody. And for surplus security there was always Fred. I didn't need to depend on any one man for bed and board or affection because there was always my dear, reliable husband. And if ever there was a threat of rejection of me during an affair, a rare event, I could turn to the 'security' of my marriage. I would drop that man so hard his balls would clank. I learned that expression from Helen. It amuses you, I see. I could then focus on the next man on my list of good prospects and he would begin chasing me."

She looked disdainful. "Men really are animals! Like dogs after a female in heat."

"They pick up your scent and go after you," I said.

"I guess I was a bitch, but never really in heat. All men want is whatever they can get, my father told me. And generally it's true. The fact that I have a husband and home rarely stopped them. I think," she said, pulling her fur sweater around her, "it only makes the chase more attractive to them."

"But what about your contribution to the chase?" I said. "You told me you usually let the man know that it was just a game not to be taken seriously."

"Not at first. At the beginning I let him think the chase is meaningful. Once he falls into the trap, I try to convince him that I want our relationship to be for amusement only. Those who agree not to take our affair seriously and want to pursue me anyway, I drop immediately. But if he becomes hooked on me, I insist it's just a game for me and should be for him too. Then I watch him fall deeper and deeper in love with me, and I have what I want."

"A squirming, pleading male, who thinks he loves you and is in great pain trying to convince you to take him seriously, like John."

"Exactly," she said, gazing sternly at me. "Exactly."

"At that moment your unconscious vengeance on your father is at full wrath," I said. "You then have him in your grip where you can crush him as you unconsciously felt you wanted to crush your father when you were a small child and even an adolescent. You choose carefully, selecting only a man vulnerable to such pain or suffering. Then you conquer him, villify and discard him, and start all over. Your need to renew your vengeance is insatiable and will remain so unless you begin to understand it and work on it. As for Fred, he is neuter gender. He's not a man, nor a husband—only a safe, controllable possession, a counterpart of you. He has his own pathology, I suspect."

She looked down for a moment. "I guess I've always known he has deeper problems than he is aware of, or is willing to face, or that I want to think about, because my needs came first."

Her anger was gone. She seemed for a moment to be with me, without affectation or malice. She looked strangely sad.

"I feel sorry for him," she said. "I know I will have to leave him some day."

"So you do have some feelings for Fred, don't you?"

"Only for the part of him which is human, I guess. You're right. The part of him that makes him a male never concerns me.

She began the next session with the same degree of anxiety and seriousness with which she ended the last session. These were the first of such reactions by her. The mobilization of these feelings was an important sign. It meant that she had the capacity to attain new and intense affects which could be developed.

"You helped me realize something when you spoke of my feeling for men last time," she said. "My feelings for women are—are stronger than I want them to be—for Louise, for other women. Yet I've never had an affair with a woman or even wanted to. What a sordid thought, to have an affair with a woman. I only like to be close to women friends because they can be trusted."

"Like Helen," I said.

Her eyes stared through me. "Too many women have complimented me on my good looks," she said. "I always laughed at them as being jealous."

"Now you realize there may be more to it than simple admiration or envy, not necessarily that Helen or Louise was overtly interested in you. I believe they're innocent of conscious sexual wishes, from your description of them. But they appealed to you because they were trustworthy. Likewise you must appeal to them for many reasons, some of them unconscious. Remember, you trusted your mother though you had contempt for her. This doesn't necessarily mean that you had an actual homosexual interest in Louise or Helen. Certain elements of such an interest are latently present in you but are insufficient to develop into overt homosexuality.

"Heterosexuality is, contrary to popular belief, not an all-or-none proposition, but a qualitative matter. You know, some men are turned on by certain types of women and not others. Many men enjoy effeminate, petite girls. Others want aggressive or mothering women, and some even desire masculine-looking, strong women. Women, too, have different tastes. A person's individual life history largely determines his feelings of preference for a given type of mate. A small group of men and women can even literally swing either way to male or female, but most people are steadfast in their choice of sexual objects insofar as gender is concerned.

"Women too, prefer males who, in their fantasies, possess some specific idealized cultural characteristics, such as a man who is the typical Hollywood good-looking, strong-male type, or the cosmopolitan intellectual type, or the fatherly, caring type, or a combination of these and other types. There can be and are enormous variations in a woman's preferences just as there are with a man's, again determined by the varying life history of the person involved.

"Yes, you trust Louise and you almost fell in love with her. But you have enough of a feeling for males to limit this, I believe—I've sensed it in you—and enough genuine gratitude toward her to prevent you from really harming her by stealing the man she loves. That's why you came to see me at this time: because you knew that your need for vengeance toward males after more than twenty years of retaliation was getting out of hand. It was about to destroy your only real friend, Louise, who in part represents your mother, whom you also resented bitterly for failing to stand up for you against your father, and for failing to cherish you as you wish she had. But part of you loved your mother as you do Louise."

I paused. "I sound as if I'm delivering a lecture today," I said.

"No," Faith said. "It makes sense to me, as if I knew it all somewhere inside of me, even before you said it."

The weeks and months went on. We researched again and again the maldevelopment of her relationships with people, reviewing the major past and present events of her life and her responses to them. New insights arose from discoveries we made in seeing these events from multiple fresh points of view. She tried to change her conscious behavior as well, based on her wish to be different.

Faith had been working with me for nearly a year now, coming in for four to five sessions a week. Her manner gradually became less flippant as she dug into her problems with a zeal unfamiliar to her. Gone was her sarcasm and intense hostility. It was apparent that there would be some drastic changes in her character structure before we were finished.

One day as I opened my waiting-room door for another patient, Faith's husband Fred leaped up at me from a chair and insisted on entering before my patient. I asked my patient to wait a few moments. I closed the door behind us.

This was not the composed, insipid man I had seen a year ago. His hair now hung uncombed over a lean, wild face. His small eyes moved rapidly in his bobbing head; his legs shifted continually. No part of him stood still.

"I've got to see you today," he said. "It's important. I feel like killing myself." He drew a revolver from his overcoat pocket. Instead of pointing the weapon at himself he pointed the black muzzle at me.

"Please." I waved my hand at the weapon in a gesture urging that he point it away from me. "I want you to come back this evening when we can talk for a while. You're terribly upset. And leave that thing at home. Or give it to a friend to keep for you. There must be other ways of handling what's bothering you."

I continued to speak quietly in an even tone, but my heart beat rapidly. I felt sweat gathering on my upper lip and forehead. I knew that his suicidal inclination could easily be converted into a homicidal one, and I feared for both our lives. I had never before been faced with an angry, agitated patient threatening me with a gun. I thought of fleeing from any scheduled meeting with him, but I knew he was not psychotic and I guessed that his reason would prevail if I could get him to talk with me. If I tried to flee from him, he would inevitably catch up with me, and it was best to avoid placing him in the role of being both angry and deceived. His imagination might then see me as the purveyor of the cuckoldry, which I guessed he had discovered at last, and which he had chosen to avoid seeing for so many years.

"Please," I repeated. "I can see you this evening at 6:15, if you will come back then."

He slowly lowered the muzzle. I heard the safety catch click on as he moved it with his thumb. He placed the revolver in his overcoat pocket. He nodded his head in agreement and left silently. Waves of heat continued to flood over my body. My shirt and coat were soaked.

There were many hours to go before 6:15 P.M. My tension mounted as the time neared, but I saw each of my patients as planned at his appointed hour. I knew that I must remain in control, despite my fears, and that I must continue to work as matter-of-factly as my fright allowed till I saw him that evening. I had long ago learned that the most advantageous approach for all people, myself included, was to carry on as usual and try to master any difficulties by facing them with insight and action.

Evening had come. I opened my door cautiously. "I hope you've left your revolver with a friend as I asked you to do," I said.

He shook his head, pointing to a lump in his overcoat. It was still in his pocket. He entered and sat down.

I thought it best that I should talk first to demonstrate some knowledge of what troubled him and to point out the fallacy in his emotional logic which I perceived held me responsible for his plight. "So you think your wife's therapy is the cause of your problem with her?"

He looked down at his feet from a large leather chair. There was a long pause. "No, no, of course not," he said thoughtfully. "I was always afraid she might someday leave me. That's why I was glad she didn't continue with her other psychiatrists. You're the only one she's really worked with. Every day for the last few months I could see her thinking about us more and more. I could feel it coming.

"We've been married twenty years, Doctor, and I don't want it to end now." He put his head down in his hands. "For twenty years I dreaded it—that she would get tired of the way we live together. I've always known it wasn't right, but I couldn't help it—or change it! And I do love her." He looked up. "We live a kind of life that we both agreed on without saying so. Now it's coming to an end."

He was describing their agreement whereby her infidelity was tolerated, even unconsciously encouraged.

Her therapy, which afforded her increasing insight into herself and into the origins of her dissatisfaction with their marriage, caused her to wish to break their nonverbal pact, a pact that included his "blindness."

In this state he, too, enjoyed her men, often suspecting who they were, participating in her affair vicariously, yet avoiding any direct homosexual contact with them. His powerful defenses, whose origins I knew nothing about, prevented him from exposure to a full awareness of his homosexual interests, which he gratified through Faith.

He still sat with his head down. I decided to acknowledge his sexual problem without foisting a painful awareness on him by stating his problem explicitly.

"It was an agreement between two people who could live no other way," I said. "Two people who still respect each other, despite their growing differences. True, those differences came out in therapy, but they were always there."

"I won't be able to take it, Doctor," he pleaded. Tears came to his eyes. "I thought of treatment for myself, too, once a long time ago. But I was afraid—afraid to face myself, because I knew it would be too tough on me. So I gave up the idea."

"You have thought of treatment, have you?"

"I even tried it—fifteen years ago and once before that. It only made things worse. I couldn't take it. Both times I quit after a few visits that made me feel rotten."

"Before you had a real chance?"

He interrupted. "She'll leave me soon, won't she, Doctor?" His face, pale and narrow, bore the look of a pleading child.

"She's spoken of it a good deal lately. I think she's serious."

"It's too much for me to take. I won't know how to handle my life if she leaves." He moved toward the door.

"Don't go. I want to talk with you more. I'm afraid you still might use the revolver on yourself."

"Don't worry, Doctor. It won't reflect on you. You did what you had to do for your patient."

He moved toward the door again.

"Please consider some psychiatric help," I repeated. "You might be surprised, if you give it a chance."

He stopped, turned around, and faced me. "I'd really come to kill you," he said in a monotone.

"I know."

"But you're not responsible. You only did what you had to. There would be no point in it." He began to weep, his face contorting into a grimace of shame and depression. He made no attempt to hide his tears.

"I'm going, Doctor. I'm sorry I caused you any trouble."

"Please," I said. "Don't go yet!"

The door shut.

I quickly phoned Faith to tell her my fears.

"I know," she said. "I've felt it coming for a long time. I tried to get him to see you or somebody else but he wouldn't."

"Do you think he really might harm himself?" I asked.

"I don't know," she said. "I've never seen him like this before. He cried tonight before he left. He didn't tell me where he was going. He said he was afraid he'd lose me, and everyone and everything he valued would be gone. Doctor Sherwood, can he really be that afraid of losing me—after all that has gone on in our supposed marriage? I thought Fred and I had such a clear understanding—I thought I knew him so well—he was always so passive and yielding to me. I could do anything I wanted, as I've always told you."

"This is a different person we're talking about, I'm afraid, Faith, not the man you've known for all these years. He knows the agreement between the two of you is about to end. Losing you for good is much different from loaning you out to another man for a night or two."

"I told him this morning," Faith confessed, "that I was going to leave him—permanently. The only way I can really develop a relationship with another person is to leave Fred and try to trust another man—to see if I could really love him—and try to work it out with him and in my analysis. I've got to while there is still time left for me to do it.

"You know, Doctor," she continued, "the man I've been telling you about, the divorced man I've known for the last year or so? I've developed such strong feelings lately—feelings I think I've never had before. I told Fred about him without telling him who he is. I told Fred I had to—I had to leave him. I want to try. It's the only way, and I think I can do it, if I work on myself, as you say. That's why Fred was so upset this morning. He knew it would come to this eventually. Both of us did."

"Where do you think Fred might have gone?" I said.

"I'm not sure—maybe his office."

"I'll meet you there," I said. "I have the address."

I beat Faith to Fred's office. When I entered the police were there. I told them who I was.

"He put the revolver into his mouth and fired upward," an officer said to me. "He's gone." Fred's body lay slumped on a chair, his hair covered with blood. "The cleaning people heard a shot and phoned for a squad car. We're waiting for the paramedics and the detectives from homicide. But he's gone. Blew his brains out."

I shook my head and left the room. I knew Faith would be along in a moment and I wanted to prevent her from seeing Fred's body. I felt a sense of deep sorrow and regret—and relief that I was still alive.

Though he was nearly a stranger to me, I wondered if treatment might have saved Fred. Society and I had failed his kind. What else might I have done, even months ago, to persuade him to see someone in therapy?

I saw Faith approaching. I waved to her to stop. I wanted her to hear it from me—to tell her as gently as possible that she had no choice but to do as she had decided to do with her life. Her planning included no such ending for Fred. Yet I wondered if this was an aspect of the vengeance against men which she unconsciously had set for herself somewhere at the onset of her marriage.

An end and a beginning, I thought, all in the same day.

In the years that followed, Faith further freed herself of her neurotic depreciation of men. The death of her husband shocked her and helped her realize that his deep and warm feelings toward her, though painful and confusing to him, were genuine. She knew now that the game she had played with him and other men was a dangerous one largely born of her relationship with her own father.

These events gave her the incentive to explore herself more intensively than ever before. She worked hard to change her feelings, as she perceived in herself a growing ability to trust and to love a man.

Chapter 13
Never-Ending Associations of a Psychiatrist-Psychoanalyst

Dear intrapsychic analyst:

I, the physician, had plucked the newborn infant raw and wet from his mother's lacerated vaginal tract and held it by its feet, butt up, to see the wonder. And then again I became the obstetrician, this time to its psyche, to tend its passage through the conflict-laden tunnels of the unconscious into the light to seek surcease of sorrow. And again I beheld it to see its wonders.

What made me think that I was entitled to a revelation—to know why that child was born, or why it existed, or why the black woman died? What gave me reason to believe that I deserved to be master of life simply because I had survived the terror of the pillboxes and the screeching deadly eighty-eights? Did I believe that because I had become the physician I dreamed of, I had also become Messiah?

"How dare you conceive and bear that baby into poverty?" I once demanded (to myself) of the young parents in the hobby-store business, with more hungry children than they could feed. Now I say to myself, "How did I dare ask such a question?"

Now, many years later, though, in my eternal search do I know something of why I lay upon my analyst's couch all those years and continue to lie there in my intrapsychic (as so many patients have lain upon mine)?

During my self-searches I beheld (or discovered in a dream): I am not the only being in the universe, an idea I entertained in the narcissism of my youth. Yet all things that exist, exist only inside of me. Within myself lie the clues to the combination locks that conceal others from me. And this too I learned: without someone meaningful to anchor me, I'm but a cinder, a speck of matter floating in the cosmos seeking desperately to be joined by others, isolated in an infinity of time and history. A dying Dannie, long since passed into the soil, taught me this. Florence's failure to love him nearly stripped him of his sweet illusion, almost left him adrift, a tiny entity afloat upon a tumult of unending loneliness in the vast kingdom of eternity.

A poet warned me long ago, but who believes poets? "Oh love, let us be true to one another," for we are all Dannies.

Even Faith the elite, Faith that former unknowable, has discovered this to be true. She seeks a man-mate whom she can both love and trust. Has she found him yet?

And this, too, I've come to know. In the infancy-childhood of a developing mind lies its chance for inner contentment. For even when one is joined unto others to touch and speak and even love, one is still alone—in his intrapsychic self. One's deepest and most constant companion will always be himself. A pacing Myrna pointed this out to me and more, the once confused Myrna who now is able to live alone in an apartment on a sandy hill above a restless sea.

Sometimes in the stillness of my empty office long after my last patient has gone, or when I awaken at home in the middle of the night, there recurs a satisfying thought: my work is a perpetual theater. Every patient is a character in a story played out before me. Some are simple tales; others, tragedies; and a few, great dramas staged before my eyes and ears alone. Bit by bit I get to know the actors in each scene, and in time I appear among the cast in my patients' thoughts and dreams.

Some patients keep in touch with me, while others survive as memories. None leaves forever. And I continue to wonder what is being written in their scripts, and what will occur in the final acts of the people who have populated my mind over the past few decades.

What has happened to all the unwanted children of all the women unthinkingly impregnated by everyone and no one?: the sons and daughters of big Jose? The big County Hospital is full of them: trampled, orphaned little ones, waiting endlessly, hoping to smile on someone till they forget how to smile, children who draw back, fearful and distrustful of everyone, and who live their lives in foster homes or homes where too few care.

Where have all these children gone, the squealing, laughing, tiny ones who threw their arms around my knees and hugged me with delight? And where have all the grown-ups gone (the children of the past) who once had been my sickly ones, the infected and the maimed, the coronaries and the cancers, the melancholy and the anxious?

The children of the black woman and her quiet husband, how much did they suffer by the loss of their mother, left alone as they were these long years with only ancient memories of her? (She fought her battle to the very edge of time to be with them.)

I kept in touch with a nursery school teacher with whom I had worked over the years and who lived near Nene's family. She informed me of the fate of Nene's mother, a woman who constantly held a hand over her face as if she were perplexed by painful thought or tried to hide part of herself from view. One rainy morning after she had dropped her daughter off at school, her car skidded over a cliff, and she was crushed. The coroner termed it an accidental death, but the teacher suspected otherwise. Nene was eight years old at the time.

During Nene's childhood, her automated father traveled a computerized schedule from city to city, selling electronic gear. His only child's number seldom came up in his retrieval system.

After his wife died, he coded Nene to be in the possession of an aunt and uncle, the only relatives who knew her. They strove desperately to be good parents to her.

At age fifteen, Nene began to disappear from their house in the evenings, returning late at night, silent about where she had been. They tried to bribe her with gifts of green jade jewelry and Indian necklaces which they owned. She had toyed with these trinkets by the hour, as a child, whenever she and her mother had visited. Nene dangled these charms in heavy layers about her thin neck, endlessly putting them on and taking them off as she stared at herself in a mirror. Still she would say nothing about where she had been, or when, and where she was going again.

Then their alarm turned to frustration. After she returned one night, they screamed and slapped her, yelling, "Nene, please! Help us help you. We want to protect you from yourself. Please, Nene, please. Tell us!"

Nene slumped to the floor, weighted down by the layers of clanking stones, and turned an expressionless face away from them in silence.

After that incident, my informant told me, Nene began to steal money and rings and more necklaces from them and from neighbors, unconsciously taking from the world what she felt was owed to her, as so many children do, wresting from everyone and anyone the pleasures denied to her during her lifetime, as she wrestled with the shadows in her mind. Her aunt and uncle grew increasingly puzzled. Finally they gave up on her.

Over the years she was shunted from one foster home to the next, still disappearing for hours when no one watched. Some say the young woman had a secret rendezvous with a spirit, others say a lover; a few believe she went to weep on her mother's grave. She lives somewhere in the wilderness of this great city, still unsmiling (I know), and no longer protected by Big Howard.

And what has become of the dozens upon dozens of other patients whom I have come to know over the years?: fearful heart patients like Harry who gained victories over their fears and those less fortunate than they? And why is Harry so poignant in my memory still? Is it because at one time I too had been overwhelmed with anxiety, abruptly thrust forth as I was in childhood to witness my grandmother's sudden disappearance from this earth, to learn too painfully the dread word "death"?

What was the essence of Harry's words? They applied to me too without his knowing it: some few face death's challenge unswervingly, even brazenly, while others face it consistently—with cowardice, like me. The brave should be grateful to us cowards. Were it not for us, they would be undistinguished and indistinguishable.

The pallid face of the Greek shoe repairman, wretched in his cancer, yet dignified, diplomatic, and scholarly to the very end, showed me how gracefully men can die. He still lies on an autopsy table in my mind, strains of Mozart clinging to his soul.

His face reminds me of an aching I had in my chest on a battlefield long, long ago: "Who will come to my funeral and what will they say? Will somebody still think of me when he awakens from his sleep in the middle of the night years from today?"

The hunched and tight-lipped Guilderman battled less well than most. He was never able to calm the rage and hurt that brewed inside him from his med school failure. Twenty years later, his marriage, too, began to fail. His atrophied self-esteem shrank even further. One day he sprang from the top of the six-story science building in which he taught biology. His body splattered on the concrete below amid his horrified students.

His widow, whom I knew from medical school days, rushed to me and flooded me with tears which overflowed from the rancor her two teenage children heaped upon her for his death.

"I hate you," her son shouted, weeping. "When you told dad you didn't love him any more, you destroyed him. When you divorced him, you ended his life."

And Faith's husband sitting in his death chair reappears to haunt me, again and again. How much did I contribute to his end by helping Faith to shake her inability to trust and love a man? It took months (or was it years?) before I could allow myself to feel that my first impulse, following my shock at seeing his body slumped and bleeding, was one of relief that he no longer stood in her way. She was free of her sick attachment, free to test her newly developed affection on another. Even now my uneasiness over the suicide of this anguished dead man begins to rise again.

Suicide! What reasonable human being has failed to consider it? I have felt in pressured moments how serenely sweet it might be if my struggles could be quelled: to be plagued no longer by the merciless thrust to prove my father's value and my own, or by the ceaseless, tormented toil of work, or by the hurt and humiliation of threatened failure, or by some momentous project gone awry, followed by the disappearance of friends who once seemed to care; to be out forever to the interminable jangling phone calls, the endless demands of people in distress; to dream of a dreamless, sleepless sleep.

And what has become of Emma and what more did she think as she spent her final days staring at a door? "You've got to face life," cackled her daughter as she fled from her mother's room, "face what it offers."

My father died and gained immortality; he saw the birth of Israel and fought its battles (through his brethren) till his very end. "Though the taunting Nazis live within me still," he said, "I have struck back through my son and that new nation, and I live as long as Israel remains alive."

My mother's Polish-Jew anxiety indirectly spawned proud, blond, sky-eyed grandchildren from the loins of an Aryan—her daughter-in-law. Lisa and she came to love each other, though my mother's ancient memories till the moment of her death never left her for a day.

I know that Obsessive Boy's parents still fight to understand him as he struggles, locked in the strange imprisonment of his cerebral torment, trying to discover how to free himself of thinking thoughts he cannot keep from thinking and touching things he cannot keep from touching.

And Belinda continues in her quest to find in life that self-comfort she had always sought to find only through others. She has continued to grow, long after our last meeting, she writes me.

And Teddy, that sweet, angry, pained fag, has kept faith with his promise to himself to live on. He labors to become the director-writer he feels he was meant to be, and he seeks, without shame, a man who can give him hope for love between them.

Was I always kind and protective—like Big Howard, a child who showed me how? And steadfast in my insights? Was I always the true physician, loving each one, my patients, and failing to despise some, even a little?

Who says I hated not at all? As I hate myself I hated some, at times.

Did I not participate in the murder of men in war? The shells and bullets I helped launch were sent with vengeance against an enemy often as innocent as I. Yet I hated them as my father had, and more. The sight of green-uniformed, bloated krauts lying dead by the roadside in droves, silently floating in the gutters, brought glee inside of me. Now I know most were only men, grown from sweet, loved children and taught to murder, much as I. I'm unable to forget the German sniper hidden in the hedgerows who toppled from my kill. Later, as he lay there, I looked into his open eyes lifted to the sky. His face half-smiled at me through clenched white teeth. His skin was clear and light. He was my age, I guessed—nineteen. (His parents still weep for him.)

And as a general practitioner did I not assume omnipotence, pretend I was a Great Gordon, and become on occasion as arrogant as D. V. Delbert, or righteous in my own belief about how to care for people? Did I not condemn a gynecologist for misdiagnosing a malignancy of the uterus in my patient, Lena Spritzger, age thirty-eight, who died as a result of that mistake? I did till one of my errors was pointed out to me; I missed the dreaded meningococcic meningitis in a child of three. And as a psychiatrist did I not think to tell Emma's daughter what she owed her mother (glad I kept my trap shut) and have contempt for some like the drunken bum, thrashing in the hall, and for George, the bloody one? I had within me the same disdain for others which Dr. Neal (that plucker of black sheep, destroyer of spirits, and lyncher of souls) had for medical students, or which Hinder of biochemistry had for all of us in his classes of long ago.

Or was I above being like that other surgeon, H. J. Visco, out for pomp or gain from my patients (or at least some part of me, rationalized by the vagaries in my field), or using displaced people like the starving women I bought in war for cigarettes and chocolate? Was I not a fool and rapist (nearly) like big Jose'?

Can I sing praises to myself that I have laid no hands where no physician's hands belong?

What's that, Hippocrates? Too many physicians have slept with their patients. Was I a saint for my chastity, while I vicariously partook of some vulvas (in my pleasure's fantasy)? Like Faith, who detailed her many affairs? Her eyes and voice (and my urges) pleaded to corrupt me, and likewise I was tempted by others: the dark-eyed Latin woman, Margarita, who begged me to bed with her. She bore the figure of a Venus with a flock of Apollos in pursuit. Was it fear of exposure alone that kept me? I pray it was more: a sense of duty, perhaps?

Then was I whore for the money I took from pained souls? At least I strove to be a saint who gave something of himself. A saintly whore may be just right for my name. For I have learned that there is none so honest or fair that he is without greed, or unnecessary pride, or petty rancor, or regret.

Regret? At one time I was full of what might have been, what should have been, and what could have been. But this is long since past, for I have obtained in medicine that which I deem to be most precious of all: I know some people called patients (with whom I spend my life) more deeply than their warmest lovers, more honestly than their closest friends, more intimately than the parents who gave them birth and nurturance (even during their childhood's candor), more touchingly than any naked infant-mother pair wrapped in each others' arms, smiling and cooing in drowsy morning's bed. And I know myself better for it.

And now I am content to know that I shall never know why that child was born, nor master life, nor know why we go on to live or die. Though my seeking continues, I have found that what I must search for, now and always, is myself.

And when I close my eyes to dream each night, blurred images appear on the retina of my inner self, and then they one by one grow clear. And this is what I see: a generous Maybelle, laughing still, and a young girl's pained face as she bears her child, and Andrew Mitchelin who lives forever in a morgue refrigerator, and Obsessive Boy, and Florence, and Faith, and a red-haired mother, and a drunken bum, and a man with a cinder in his eye, and Belinda, who is smiling now, and Teddy, and Harry, and Dannie, and Myrna, and me.